PocketRadiologist®
Breast
Top 100 Diagnoses

Specialties included in the PocketRadiologist® series

Abdominal, Top 100 Diagnoses

Brain, Top 100 Diagnoses

Cardiac, Top 100 Diagnoses

Chest, Top 100 Diagnoses

Head & Neck, Top 100 Diagnoses

Musculoskeletal, Top 100 Diagnoses

Obstetrics, Top 100 Diagnoses

Pediatrics, Top 100 Diagnoses

PedsNeuro, Top 100 Diagnoses

Spine, Top 100 Diagnoses

Temporal Bone, Top 100 Diagnoses

Vascular, Top 100 Diagnoses

and

Interventional, Top 100 Procedures

PocketRadiologist®
Breast
Top 100 Diagnoses

Robyn L Birdwell MD
Associate Professor of Radiology
Director, Radiology Residency Program
Stanford University Medical Center
Stanford, California

Elizabeth A Morris MD
Assistant Professor of Radiology
Weill Medical College of Cornell University
Assistant Attending Radiologist
Memorial Sloan-Kettering Cancer Center
New York City, New York

Shih-chang Wang MD FRANZCR
Head, Department of Diagnostic Radiology
National University of Singapore
Department of Diagnostic Imaging
National University Hospital
Singapore

Brett T Parkinson MD
Imaging Director Breast Care Services
Intermountain Health Care
Adjunct Assistant Professor of Radiology
University of Utah School of Medicine
Salt Lake City, Utah

With 200 drawings and radiographic images

Drawings:	Lane R Bennion MS
	Richard Coombs MS
Image Editing:	Melissa Petersen
	Danielle Morris
	Ming Q Huang MD
	Cassie Dearth
Medical Text Editing:	Richard H Wiggins III MD

 W. B. SAUNDERS COMPANY
An Elsevier Science Company

AMIRSYS™

AMIRSYS™

A medical reference publishing company

First Edition

First Printing: July 2003

Composition by Amirsys Inc, Salt Lake City, Utah

Printed by K/P Corporation, Salt Lake City, Utah

ISBN: 0-7216-0078-6

Preface

The **PocketRadiologist** series is an innovative, quick reference designed to deliver succinct, up-to-date information to practicing professionals "at the point of service." As close as your pocket, world-renowned authors write each title in the series. These experts have designated the "top 100" diagnoses or interventional procedures in every major body area, bulleted the most essential facts, and offered high-resolution imaging to illustrate each topic. Selected references are included for further review. Full color anatomic-pathologic computer graphics model many of the actual diseases.

Each **PocketRadiologist** title follows an identical format. The same information is in the same place - every time - and takes you quickly from key facts to imaging findings, differential diagnosis, pathology, pathophysiology, and relevant clinical information. The interventional modules give you the essentials and "how-tos" of important procedures, including pre- and post-procedure checklists, common problems and complications.

PocketRadiologist titles are available in both print and hand-held PDA formats. Currently available modules feature Brain, Head and Neck, Orthopaedic (Musculoskeletal) Imaging, Pediatrics, Spine, Chest, Cardiac, Vascular, Abdominal Imaging and Interventional Radiology. 2003 topics that will round out the PocketRadiologist series include Obstetrics, Gynecologic Imaging, Breast, Temporal Bone, Pediatric Neuroradiology and Emergency Imaging.

Anne G Osborn MD
Executive Vice President
Editor-in-Chief, Amirsys Inc

H Ric Harnsberger MD
Chairman and CEO, Amirsys Inc

Notice and Disclaimer

The information in this product ("Product") is provided as a reference for use by licensed medical professionals and no others. It does not and should not be construed as any form of medical diagnosis or professional medical advice on any matter. Receipt or use of this Product, in whole or in part, does not constitute or create a doctor-patient, therapist-patient, or other healthcare professional relationship between Amirsys Inc. ("Amirsys") and any recipient. This Product may not reflect the most current medical developments, and Amirsys makes no claims, promises, or guarantees about accuracy, completeness, or adequacy of the information contained in or linked to the Product. The Product is not a substitute for or replacement of professional medical judgment. Amirsys and its affiliates, authors, contributors, partners, and sponsors disclaim all liability or responsibility for any injury and/or damage to persons or property in respect to actions taken or not taken based on any and all Product information.

In the cases where drugs or other chemicals are prescribed, readers are advised to check the Product information currently provided by the manufacturer of each drug to be administered to verify the recommended dose, the method and duration of administration, and contraindications. It is the responsibility of the treating physician relying on experience and knowledge of the patient to determine dosages and the best treatment for the patient.

To the maximum extent permitted by applicable law, Amirsys provides the Product AS IS AND WITH ALL FAULTS, AND HEREBY DISCLAIMS ALL WARRANTIES AND CONDITIONS, WHETHER EXPRESS, IMPLIED OR STATUTORY, INCLUDING BUT NOT LIMITED TO, ANY (IF ANY) IMPLIED WARRANTIES OR CONDITIONS OF MERCHANTABILITY, OF FITNESS FOR A PARTICULAR PURPOSE, OF LACK OF VIRUSES, OR ACCURACY OR COMPLETENESS OF RESPONSES, OR RESULTS, AND OF LACK OF NEGLIGENCE OR LACK OF WORKMANLIKE EFFORT. ALSO, THERE IS NO WARRANTY OR CONDITION OF TITLE, QUIET ENJOYMENT, QUIET POSSESSION, CORRESPONDENCE TO DESCRIPTION OR NON-INFRINGEMENT, WITH REGARD TO THE PRODUCT. THE ENTIRE RISK AS TO THE QUALITY OF OR ARISING OUT OF USE OR PERFORMANCE OF THE PRODUCT REMAINS WITH THE READER.

Amirsys disclaims all warranties of any kind if the Product was customized, repackaged or altered in any way by any third party.

PocketRadiologist®
Breast
Top 100 Diagnoses

The diagnoses in this book are divided into 9 sections in the following order:

BIRADS™
Benign Lesions
Risk Lesions
Malignancies
The Male Breast
Post-Op Benign
Post-Op Cancer
Hormone Changes
Procedures

Table of Contents

Table of Contents

The Male Breast

Post-Op Benign

Table of Contents

Post-Op Cancer

Hormone Changes

Procedures

PocketRadiologist®
Breast
Top 100 Diagnoses

BIRADS™

Masses

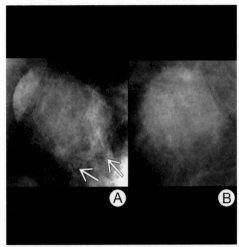

(A) Oval well-circumscribed mass with < 25% of margin obscured by overlying tissue (arrows) in a 35-year-old. Ultrasound = cyst. (B) 34-year-old with palpable mass seen on mammogram as a round mass with indistinct margins suggesting infiltration into surrounding tissue. Biopsy = infiltrating ductal carcinoma.

Key Facts
- BIRADS™ mammographic definition: Space occupying lesion seen in two different projections
  - A possible mass seen in only one projection = "density"
- BIRADS ultrasound definition: Occupies space and should be seen in two projections
- BIRADS MRI definition: A three-dimensional space-occupying lesion
  - Separate definition = focus or foci of enhancement
    - Tiny spot(s) of enhancement too small to be characterized
    - No clear mass on precontrast images
    - Synonyms: UBO, unidentified bright objects; IEL, incidental enhancing lesions
  - Separate definitions for non-mass enhancement patterns

Imaging Findings
Mammography Findings
- Shape
  - Round
  - Oval
  - Lobular
  - Irregular
- Margins
  - Circumscribed
  - Microlobulated
  - Obscured
    - Masked by surrounding breast tissue
  - Indistinct
  - Spiculated
- Density

3

Masses

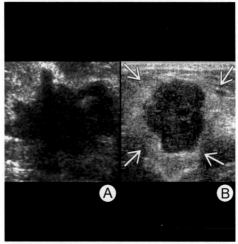

Sonographic images of infiltrating ductal carcinomas. (A) Hypoechoic mass has an irregular shape, is not parallel to skin, & has spiculated margins & posterior acoustic shadowing. (B) Irregular hypoechoic mass is not parallel to skin, has fairly smooth margins with thick rim (arrows), & posterior acoustic enhancement.

- o Higher than surrounding tissue
- o Equal
- o Low
- o Fat-containing
  - ▪ Part or all of the lesion

Ultrasound Findings
- Shape
  - o Oval
  - o Round
  - o Irregular
- Orientation (unique to ultrasound)
  - o Parallel to skin line
  - o Not parallel to skin line
- Margins
  - o Circumscribed
  - o Indistinct
  - o Angular
  - o Microlobulated
  - o Spiculated
- Lesion boundary
  - o No perceptible rim or thin rim
  - o Thick rim
- Internal echogenicity as compared with breast fat
  - o Anechoic
  - o Hyperechoic
  - o Complicated cyst
    - ▪ Mobile low level echoes
    - ▪ Fluid-debris level
  - o Complex

Masses

  - o Hypoechoic
- Posterior acoustic features
  - o No effect
  - o Enhancement
  - o Shadowing
  - o Combined enhancement and shadowing

Gadolinium Enhanced MR Findings for Focal Enhancement (Mass)
- Shape
  - o Round or oval
  - o Lobulated
  - o Irregular
- Margins
  - o Smooth
  - o Irregular
  - o Spiculated
- Internal enhancement
  - o Homogeneous
  - o Heterogeneous
  - o Rim
  - o Dark internal septations
  - o Enhancing internal septations
  - o Central
- Non-mass enhancement patterns
  - o Linear (not a duct)
  - o Ductal
  - o Segmental
  - o Regional
  - o Diffuse
- Non-mass internal enhancement
  - o Homogeneous
  - o Heterogeneous
  - o Stippled Punctate
  - o Clumped

Differential Diagnosis
Imaging and Clinical Findings Dictate Level of Suspicion

Pathology
General
- Likelihood of malignancy may be predicted on imaging
  - o With increasing irregularity of shape and margins
  - o With intense enhancement on MRI

Clinical Issues
Presentation
- Cancers may be clinically or image-detected

Selected References
1.   Ikeda DM: Progress report from the american college of radiology breast MR imaging lexicon committee. Breast MR imaging. Clin No Am 9:295-302, 2001
2.   Mendelson EB et al: Toward a standardized breast ultrasound lexicon, BIRADS: Ultrasound. Semin Roentgenol 3:217-25, 2001
3.   ACR Illustrated BIRADS™, 3rd ed. 9-52, 1998

Calcifications

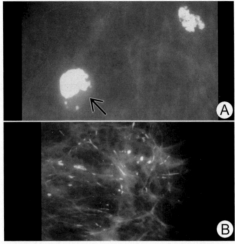

Two benign types of calcifications. (A) Note "popcorn" calcifications associated with involuting fibroadenomas. A portion of soft-tissue mass can be seen in lower left (arrow). (B) Secretory calcifications. Note linear branching but coarse nature of these benign intra-or periductal calcifications secondary to plasma cell mastitis.

Key Facts
- BIRADS™ mammographic definition
  - Calcification types
    - Benign
    - Intermediate concern
    - Higher probability of malignancy
- BIRADS ultrasound definition: Limited benefit for calcifications
- BIRADS MRI definition: No specific enhancement characteristics

Imaging Findings
Mammography Findings
- Benign (> 0.5 mm)
  - Skin (dermal)
    - Polygonal-shaped
    - Lucent or umbilicated centers
    - Seen in skin on tangential x-ray image
  - Vascular
    - Parallel continuous or discontinuous tracks
    - Few branch points (typically the ductal system arborizes more frequently than do vessels in the breast)
  - Coarse "popcorn"
    - Within involuting fibroadenoma
  - Rod-like ("cigar" shaped)
    - > 1 mm diameter
    - Follow ductal distribution
    - Secondary to plasma cell mastitis or duct ectasia
  - Round
    - Variable size
    - Smooth margins

Calcifications

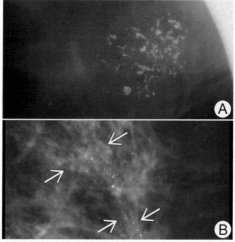

Calcifications. (A) Demonstrates a cluster of linear and linear-branching calcifications. (B) Pleomorphic calcifications in a linear-branching distribution (arrows). Both cases proved to be ductal carcinoma in situ at biopsy.

- "Punctate" < 0.5 mm
- Form in lobule acini
  - o Lucent-centered
    - Round or oval
    - Fat necrosis and calcified duct debris
  - o "Eggshell"
    - Thin, calcified, spherical surface
    - Oil cysts
  - o Milk-of-calcium
    - Particulate calcium in micro-cysts
    - Smudgy appearance on CC mammogram
    - Linear or meniscus form on lateral mammogram
  - o Suture
  - o Dystrophic
    - Irregular shape
    - > 0.5 mm
    - Lucent centers
    - Found in irradiated or traumatized breast
- Intermediate concern
  - o Amorphous, indistinct
    - Round
    - Flake-shaped
    - Small or hazy
- Malignant characteristics (< 0.5 mm)
  - o Fine linear
    - May branch
    - Within ducts
    - "Casting type"
  - o Pleomorphic
    - Variations in forms and sizes

Calcifications

- o Granular
  - ▪ Irregular margins
- Distribution modifiers
  - o Clustered
    - ▪ Multiple calcifications in small tissue volume
    - ▪ May be present with benign or malignant processes
  - o Linear
    - ▪ May have branch points
    - ▪ Suggests ductal origin
    - ▪ Suggests possible malignant process
  - o Segmental
    - ▪ Triangular arrangement directed toward nipple
    - ▪ Suggests ductal system involvement
    - ▪ Suggests possible malignant process
  - o Regional
    - ▪ Large area involved
    - ▪ Suggests a benign process
  - o Diffuse (scattered)
    - ▪ Random distribution throughout one or both breasts
    - ▪ Suggests a benign process

Ultrasound Findings
- Poorly characterized
- If present
  - o Macrocalcifications
    - ▪ > 0.5 mm
    - ▪ May shadow if very large
  - o Microcalcifications
    - ▪ Outside of a mass difficult to discern
    - ▪ Within a mass, may be seen as bright reflectors

MR Findings
- T1 C+
  - o No enhancement specific to calcifications
  - o Large deposits may show signal void on noncontrast imaging
  - o Calcified tumors may demonstrate abnormal enhancement patterns

Differential Diagnosis
Imaging and Clinical Findings Dictate Level of Suspicion for Biopsy Recommendation

Pathology
General
- Malignancy more common with suspicious morphologic and distribution patterns

Clinical Issues
Presentation
- Cancers may be clinically or image-detected

Selected References
1. Ikeda DM: Progress report from the American college of radiology breast MR imaging lexicon committee. Breast MR Imaging Clin No Am 9:295-302, 2001
2. Mendelson EB et al: Toward a standardized breast ultrasound lexicon, BIRADS: Ultrasound. Semin Roentgenol 3:217-25, 2001
3. ACR Illustrated BIRADS™, 3rd ed. 9-52, 1998

Special Cases

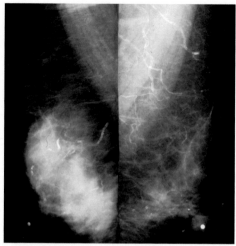

Special cases. MLO mammogram in asymptomatic 80-year-old woman intermittently taking hormonal replacement shows marked asymmetry of breast tissue with more tissue present on right. Random ultrasound-guided core biopsies revealed normal breast tissue & mammogram has now been stable X 4 years.

Key Facts
- BIRADS™ mammographic definition: Findings not categorized as masses or calcifications
  - Architectural distortion
  - Tubular density
  - Intramammary lymph node
  - Asymmetric breast tissue
  - Focal asymmetric density
- BIRADS ultrasound definition: Those cases with a unique diagnosis or findings
  - Mass in or on skin
  - Foreign body
  - Intramammary lymph nodes
  - Axillary lymph nodes
  - Vascularity

Imaging Findings
<u>Mammography Findings</u>
- Architectural distortion
  - No visible mass
  - Disruption of normal tissue planes
    - Tethering
    - Tenting
    - Spiculations
  - May represent benign or malignant changes
    - Scar
    - Carcinoma
- Tubular density (single dilated duct)

Special Cases

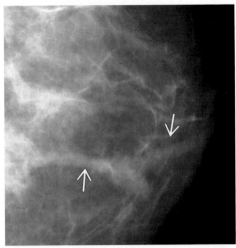

Spot mammographic image demonstrates a single dilated duct (arrows). The clinical setting was an asymptomatic woman with stable mammograms over the past 6 years. No biopsy was performed.

- o Suspicious
  - ▪ Associated with clinical findings
  - ▪ Differentiate from Mondor's disease
  - ▪ Associated with other mammographic findings
  - ▪ Papilloma
  - ▪ Uncommon presentation of ductal carcinoma in situ (DCIS)
- Intramammary lymph node
  - o Reniform fat-containing mass
  - o < 1 cm
  - o Lateral breast
  - o May be multiple
- Asymmetric breast tissue
  - o No focal mass
  - o No architectural distortion
  - o No worrisome calcifications
  - o Nonpalpable
- Focal asymmetric density
  - o Similar on both mammographic projections
  - o Lacks borders
  - o Not a true mass
  - o May represent island of tissue

Ultrasound Findings
- Mass in or on skin
- Foreign body
- Intramammary lymph node
  - o 0.3-1.5 cm
  - o Hypoechoic oval mass with internal echogenicity
    - ▪ Lymphoidal tissue surrounding fat
    - ▪ Presence of fat does not exclude tumor involvement
  - o Enlargement secondary to benign and malignant processes

Special Cases

- Lymphoid hyperplasia
  - Sinus histiocytosis
  - Inflammatory conditions
  - Lymphoma
  - Metastatic tumor
- Axillary lymph nodes
  - Size quite variable
  - Hypoechoic oval mass with internal echogenicity
    - Lymphoidal tissue surrounding fat
    - Presence of fat does not exclude tumor involvement
  - Enlargement secondary to benign and malignant processes
    - Lymphoid hyperplasia
    - Sinus histiocytosis
    - Inflammatory conditions
    - Lymphoma
    - Metastatic tumor
- Vascularity
  - None
  - Present in lesion
  - Present immediately adjacent to lesion
  - Increased in surrounding tissue

Differential Diagnosis
Imaging and Clinical Findings Dictate Level of Suspicion for Biopsy
Recommendation

Pathology
General
- Likelihood of malignancy may be predicted on imaging
  - With increasing irregularity of shape and margins
  - With intense enhancement on MRI
  - With associated clinical findings

Clinical Issues
Presentation
- Cancers may be clinically or image detected

Selected References
1. Mendelson E et al: Toward a standardized breast ultrasound lexicon, BIRADS: Ultrasound. Semin Roentgenol 36:217-25, 2001
2. Rosen PP: Breast pathology: Diagnosis by needle core biopsy. Lippincott Williams & Wikins, Philadelphia PA; Chapter24, 247-50, 1999
3. ACR Illustrated BIRADS™, 3rd ed. 127-41, 1998

Associated Findings

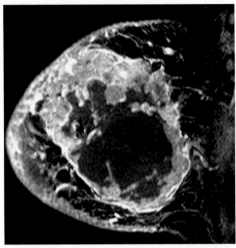

Associated findings. The gadolinium-enhanced fat-suppressed sagittal MRI image shows a large, intensely enhancing, invasive ductal carcinoma with central necrosis and associated diffuse skin thickening. The skin enhancement immediately adjacent to the anterior tumor margin suggests direct tumor involvement.

Key Facts
- BIRADS™ mammographic definition: Characteristics added to descriptions of masses and calcification
- BIRADS ultrasound definition: Mass effect on surrounding tissue
- BIRADS MRI definition: Findings associated with abnormal enhancement patterns
- May stand alone as findings without other abnormalities

Imaging Findings
Mammography Findings
- Skin retraction
  - Pulled in toward chest wall
- Nipple retraction
  - Inverted
- Skin thickening
  - Focal
  - Diffuse
- Trabecular thickening
  - Thickened, hazy, fibrous septae
- Skin lesion
  - Distinguished from parenchymal lesion
- Axillary adenopathy
  - Soft-tissue masses
  - Not fatty replaced
  - Nonspecific
    - Hyperplasia
    - Tumor infiltration
- Architectural distortion
  - Interruption of normal tissue planes associated with another finding
- Calcifications

Associated Findings

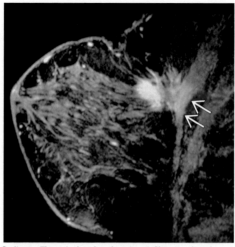

Associated findings. The spiculated, enhancing, infiltrating ductal carcinoma shows associated pectoralis muscle enhancement (arrows). The muscle was involved with tumor at surgery.

- o Within or adjacent to another finding

Ultrasound Findings
- Ducts
  - o Abnormal caliber
  - o Abnormal arborization
- Cooper's ligament changes
  - o Straightening
  - o Thickening
- Edema
  - o Increased echogenicity of tissue around focal finding
  - o Reticulation including angular hypoechoic lines
- Architectural distortion
- Skin thickening/irregularity
  - o > 2 mm
- Skin retraction

MR Findings
- Skin retraction
  - o Enhancement
    - Recent surgery
    - Trauma
    - Tumor
  - o No enhancement
    - Prior surgery
    - Prior radiation therapy
    - Prior trauma with scarring
- Nipple retraction
  - o Enhancement
    - Nipple normally enhances
    - Underlying tumor

- Skin thickening
  - Enhancement
    - Recent surgery
    - Trauma
    - Tumor
  - No enhancement
    - Prior surgery
    - Prior radiation therapy
    - Prior trauma with scarring
- Edema
- Lymphadenopathy
  - Enlarged, round-shaped lymph nodes with loss of fatty hila
  - Enhancement
    - Hyperplastic
    - Tumor infiltration
- Pectoralis muscle invasion
  - Enhancement extending into adjacent pectoralis muscle
- Chest wall invasion
  - Enhancement extending into ribs or intercostal spaces
- Hematoma/seroma
  - Typically seen following recent surgery
  - Fluid-filled, smoothly marginated cavities
    - Hypointense, smooth, thin rim enhancement
    - Thick, clumped rim or surrounding enhancement may = residual tumor
  - Seromas
    - Hyperintense on T2WI
  - Hematomas
    - Hyper- or hypointense on T1WI
    - Depends on age and oxygenation of blood products
- Abnormal signal void
  - Absence of signal due to artifact

Differential Diagnosis
Findings Require Close Scrutiny to Differentiate Benign From Malignant

Pathology
General
- Likelihood of malignancy may be predicted on imaging
  - With increasing irregularity of shape and margins
  - With intense enhancement and early washout or "de-enhancement" on MRI

Clinical Issues
Presentation
- Cancers may be clinically or image detected

Selected References
1. Mendelson E et al: BIRADS: Ultrasound. Seminars Roentgen 36:217-25, 2001
2. Morris EA et al: Evaluation of pectoralis major muscle in patients with posterior breast tumors on breast MR images; early experience. Radiology 214:67-72, 2000
3. ACR Illustrated BIRADS™, 3rd ed. 143-62, 1998

PocketRadiologist®
Breast
Top 100 Diagnoses

BENIGN LESIONS

Abscess

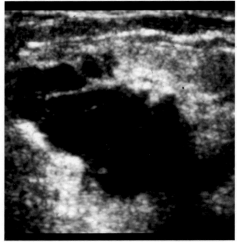

Abscess. Lactating 33-y/o with an edematous, erythematous, warm left breast & a focal painful mass in upper outer quadrant. Sonography shows a complex, 2.7 cm, irregular, hypoechoic & anechoic mass with surrounding echogenic findings 2° edema. If resolved after 2 US guided aspirations & systemic antibiotics.

Key Facts
- Synonym: Focal breast infection
- Definition: Localized pus collection within the breast tissue
- Classic imaging appearance: Hypoechoic, irregular, complex sonographic mass with surrounding increased echogenecity (edema)
  - Ill-defined, noncalcified mammographic mass
  - Mammography not often performed in younger women with the constellation suggesting infection
- Other key facts
  - Typically in lactating women
  - Staphylococcus, streptococcus most common agents
  - Can occur as a delayed infection in post-lumpectomy seroma cavities

Imaging Findings
Mammography Findings
- Pain may limit use of mammography
- Ill-defined, noncalcified mass
- Lateral view may show fluid/debris level
- Variable margin characteristics
  - Ill-defined
  - Irregular
  - Spiculated

Ultrasound Findings
- May be most beneficial imaging modality
- Young age supports value and use of ultrasound
- Hypoechoic mass
- Variable margin characteristics
  - Irregular
  - Circumscribed
  - Spiculated

Abscess

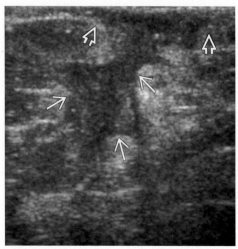

Abscess. 36-year-old with 7 month history of a right abscess cavity refractory to conservative treatment. Two surgical debridement procedures were required. The irregular, hypoechoic cavity (arrows) is seen to extend to the skin surface (open arrows).

- May have a fluid/debris level
- Air may be present within abscess cavity
  - Bright specular reflectors

MR Findings
- Conventional imaging usually sufficient
- Edema presents as high signal on T2WI
- Abscess cavity may enhance

Differential Diagnosis

Inflammatory Carcinoma
- Can mimic infectious process
  - May appear to respond to antibiotics
  - May lead to delay in diagnosis
- Skin biopsy is diagnostic
  - May have false negative results

Lactational Mastitis
- Diffuse infection may harbor a focal abscess
- Infectious agent enters through nipple
- Systemic or local treatment based on cultured agent

Nonlactational Mastitis
- Various agents
  - Fungal
  - Parasitic
  - Mycobacterial
  - Viral
  - Cat scratch disease
- Systemic or local treatment based on cultured agent

Subareolar Abscess
- Nonlactating premenopausal women

- Duct obstruction
- Duct excision may be required

Pathology
<u>General</u>
- Bacterial entry via nipple
  - o Stasis and duct obstruction contribute
- Etiology-Pathogenesis
  - o Staphylococcus more localized and invasive
  - o Streptococcus more diffuse
    - Cellulitis
    - Abscesses in advanced cases
<u>Gross Pathologic, Surgical Features</u>
- Focal mass
- Inflammation
<u>Microscopic Features</u>
- Leukocyte count > 10^6
- Bacterial count > 10^3
- Mixed acute and chronic inflammation
- May have fat necrosis

Clinical Issues
<u>Presentation</u>
- Painful focal or diffuse skin thickening and edema
- Focal abscess may present as painful mass
  - o Surrounded by diffuse edema and inflammation
<u>Natural History</u>
- May resolve
- Typically require local or systemic treatment
<u>Treatment</u>
- Aspiration of abscess cavity to diagnose infectious agent
- Exclude malignancy
- Sonographic guidance often very helpful for diagnosis and treatment
  - o Cavities < 3 cm may be completely evacuated with aspiration
  - o Cavities > 3 cm likely require indwelling catheter drainage
  - o Complex cavities also may require indwelling catheter drainage
- Systemic antibiotics based on cultured agent
- Surgical excision required for refractory cases

Selected References
1. Ellis RS: Percutaneous breast abscess management: Ultrasound-guided drainage. Radiology 225(P):683, 2002
2. Rosen PP: Rosen's breast pathology. Lippincott Williams & Wikins, Philadelphia PA; Chapter 4, 65-75, 2001
3. Bassett LW et al: Diagnosis of diseases of the breast. Philadelphia: WB Saunders Co; Chapter 25, 382-5, 1997

Axillary Breast Tissue

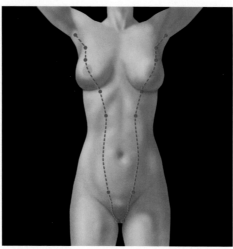

Drawing demonstrates the bilateral "milk lines" that develop from the base of the primitive forelimb (the axillary area) to the base of the primitive hindlimb bud (the inguinal area). Aberrant breast tissue can be found anywhere along this "milk line" with rare reports of the development of breast carcinoma.

Key Facts
- Synonym: Ectopic breast tissue
- Definition
  - Supernumerary breast tissue
    - Persistence of mammary ridge tissue
    - May have associated nipple and/or areolar complex
  - Aberrant or accessory breast tissue
    - Separate mammary glandular parenchyma
    - Close to usual anatomic extent of the breast
- Other key facts
  - Normal appearing breast tissue in the axilla
  - Aberrant breast tissue more common in left axilla
  - Rare reports of cancer development

Imaging Findings
Mammography Findings
- Breast tissue seen in the axilla on mediolateral oblique (MLO) view
  - Accessory nipples may be imaged
Ultrasound Findings
- Indistinguishable from breast tissue
MR Findings
- Characteristics of breast tissue
- Enhancing lesions should be assessed as in orthotopic breast
Imaging Recommendations
- No further recommendations unless imaging or clinical abnormality present

Axillary Breast Tissue

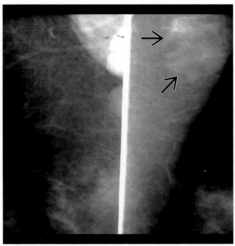

Axillary breast tissue. A small amount of normal-appearing breast tissue is seen within the left axilla (arrows). Properly positioned mediolateral oblique mammographic views should attempt to view as much of axillary region as possible in order to include possible accessory axillary tissue.

Differential Diagnosis
<u>Axillary Nodes</u>
- Discrete masses with convex margins and fatty hila
- Margins may be less discrete if enlarged or inflamed

<u>Lipoma</u>
- Circumscribed, well-defined masses of mature adipose tissue
- Axillary glandular tissue may be partly or entirely replaced by fat
  - May give clinical impression of lipoma

Pathology
<u>General</u>
- General Path Comments
  - Cytologic findings depend on tissue developmental state
- Embryology-Anatomy
  - Breast tissue same ectodermal origin as skin glands
  - Mammary ridge develops along the "milk line"
    - Base of the forelimb bud (primitive axilla) upper extent
    - Medial base of hindlimb bud (primitive inguinal area) lower extent
  - Normal development limits persistence of mammary ridge tissue
    - Middle segment of upper 1/3 adjacent to sternum
    - Posterior tissue may extend into the axilla (tail of Spence)
  - Mammary ridge tissue may persist anywhere along the "milk line"
  - Supernumerary nipples (polythelia) located on anterior chest
    - Above or below orthotopic breast
  - Benign tumors reported in ectopic locations
    - Adenomas in axilla and vulva
    - Develop during pregnancy and lactation
    - Fibroadenomas in vulva
    - Papillomas and apocrine metaplasia

Axillary Breast Tissue

o   Carcinoma reported most frequent site = axilla
  ▪   Occurs in vulva and other ectopic sites

<u>Microscopic Features</u>
• Duct and lobular mammary structures

Clinical Issues
<u>Presentation</u>
• Accessory axillary tissue may be palpable
• Accessory nipples visible
• Physiologic changes may occur
  o   Menstrual cycle
  o   Pregnancy
  o   Postpartum
    ▪   Swelling
    ▪   Pain
    ▪   Lactation when nipple present

<u>Treatment</u>
• None

Selected References
1.   Rosen PP: Rosen's breast pathology. Lippincott Williams & Wikins, Philadelphia PA; Chapter 2, 25-6, 2001
2.   Irvin WP, et al: Primary breast carcinoma of the vulva: A case report and literature review. Gynecolog Oncol 73:155-9, 1999
3.   Evans DM et al: Carcinoma of the axillary breast. J Surg Oncol 59:190-5, 1995

Breast Cyst

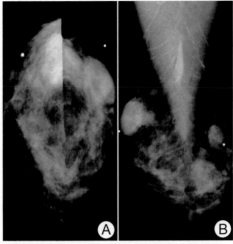

Breast cyst. 69-year-old woman with palpable lumps in both breasts. (A & B) Four-view mammogram: Bilateral, well-circumscribed, partially obscured masses. All were shown to be cysts on follow-up ultrasound.

Key Facts
- Definition
  - Simple: Fluid-filled round to oval structure which is lined by epithelium
  - Complicated: Otherwise simple cysts but with low-level homogeneous echoes
  - Complex: Cyst which on ultrasound displays thin septations, posterior acoustic shadowing, or intracystic mass
- Most common mass in the female breast
  - Peak prevalence age 35-50
  - Can occur at any age
- May be solitary or multiple
- Cannot distinguish from solid mass on mammography
  - Ultrasound useful for cystic-solid differentiation
- Simple cysts have no malignant potential
- Malignancy rate for complex cysts 0.3%
- May proliferate under estrogenic stimulation
- Size may fluctuate with menstrual cycle
  - Maximum size premenstrual phase
- Rare in males

Imaging Findings
Mammography Findings
- Well-circumscribed mass
  - Usually round or oval and of low to medium density
  - Occasionally lobulated
- Rim or eggshell calcification
  - Calcified cyst wall
Ultrasound Findings
- Well-circumscribed, thin-walled mass

Breast Cyst

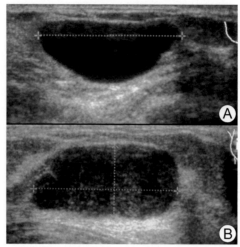

Breast cyst. (A) Well-circumscribed, oval anechoic mass with posterior acoustic enhancement. (B) Complicated cyst. Well-circumscribed hypoechoic mass with internal echoes demonstrating swirling motion on real-time imaging. Cyst resolved completely with aspiration.

- o Round or oval
- Usually anechoic
- Occasionally hypoechoic (complicated cyst)
  - o Echoes due to internal debris (proteinacious fluid)
    - ▪ May demonstrate motion on real-time imaging
- Other causes of internal echoes
  - o Blood
  - o Cellular debris
  - o Infection
  - o Cholesterol crystals
  - o Often difficult to distinguish from solid lesion
- Lateral edge refraction
  - o Echo attenuation distal to lateral margins
- Flattening observed with transducer compression
  - o Not observed with solid masses
- High-resolution, high-frequency transducer required for diagnosis
  - o 7.5 megahertz or higher (10 MHz or higher suggested but not required)
  - o Can detect cysts as small as 2-3 mm

MR Findings
- T1 (MRI not usually indicated simply to rule out cysts)
  - o T1C-
    - ▪ Smooth contour, low-signal intensity
  - o T1C+
    - ▪ No enhancement
- T2WI
  - o Smooth contour
  - o Extremely high, homogenous signal intensity

Breast Cyst

<u>Imaging Recommendations</u>
- Mammography and ultrasound
  - Ultrasound 96-100% accurate

Differential Diagnosis
<u>Fibroadenoma</u>
- Occurs in younger age group
- Solid on ultrasound
<u>Well-Circumscribed Carcinoma</u>
<u>Lymph Node</u>
- Partial fatty replacement on mammography
- Solid mass on ultrasound
  - Echogenic center (fat)

Pathology
<u>General</u>
- Etiology-Pathogenesis
  - Thought to arise from obstructed ducts
    - Dilatation of terminal ducts within lobules
    - Imbalance between secretion and absorption
<u>Gross Pathologic, Surgical Features</u>
- Rounded contour
- Bluish color ("blue-domed" cyst)
- Size: Microscopic up to 5-6 cm in diameter
<u>Microscopic Features</u>
- Dilated lobular acini
- Usually lined by single or double layer of cuboidal epithelium

Clinical Issues
<u>Presentation</u>
- Soft, fluctuant, freely movable on physical exam
  - Firm if under tension
- Tender
- Often asymptomatic
  - Detected on screening mammography
- May develop or regress rapidly
<u>Natural History</u>
- May enlarge, persist several years, or resolve spontaneously
<u>Treatment</u>
- Aspiration if painful or equivocal on imaging
  - Should be performed under ultrasound guidance
  - Routine cytology not indicated for non-bloody fluid
  - Residual mass
    - Biopsy
- Complex cyst
  - Intracystic mass
    - Biopsy

Selected References
1. Berg WA, et al. Cystic lesions of the breast: Sonographic-pathologic correlation. Radiology 227:183-91, 2003
2. Venta, LA et al: Management of complex breast cysts. AJR 173:1331-6, 1999
3. Smith, DN: Impalpable breast cysts: Utility of cytologic examination Of fluid obtained with radiologically guided aspiration. Radiology 204:149-51, 1997

Breast Edema

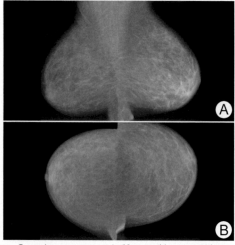

Breast edema. Screening mammogram in 60-year-old woman with congestive heart failure. Note overall increased density in fatty tissue with trabecular coarsening and skin thickening. (A) Bilateral MLO view. (B) Bilateral CC view.

Key Facts
- Definition: Abnormal accumulation of extracellular fluid in the interstices of the breast tissue
- Accompanied by skin thickening
  - Normal skin thickness 2 mm or less
  - Skin normally thicker inferiorly and medially
- Other key facts
  - Secondary to both benign and malignant causes
  - Decreases sensitivity and diagnostic value of mammography
    - Breast less compressible
    - Increased density may obscure other findings
  - May be bilateral or unilateral

Imaging Findings
Mammography Findings
- Increased density
  - Diffuse
- Skin thickening
  - Contributes to overall increased density
    - Superimposition of two layers of skin
- Affected breast may be enlarged
- Reticular pattern
  - Increased prominence of interstitial markings
Ultrasound Findings
- Disruption of normal breast echotexture
  - Variable parenchymal echo patterns
- Skin thickening
  - Increased separation of superficial and deep echogenic lines of skin complex (delineates dermis)
  - Increased echogenicity of dermis

Breast Edema

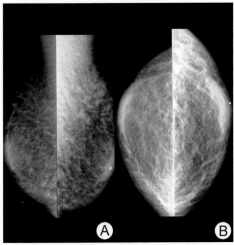

Breast edema. 70-year-old man with congestive heart failure came for breast evaluation with the complaint of enlarging breasts. (A) MLO and (B) CC views demonstrate trabecular coarsening, overall increased breast density, and skin thickening (best seen along dependent breast surfaces).

- Band-like, linear, hypoechoic structures
  - Interstitial fluid collections
  - Non-ductal distribution

Imaging Recommendations
- Mammography
- Ultrasound as dictated by mammographic or clinical findings

Differential Diagnosis

Inflammatory Breast Carcinoma (IBC)
- Unilateral
  - Bilateral IBC extremely rare
- Clinical findings suggestive of diagnosis
  - Enlarged, tender, firm breast
  - Erythema, edema and skin thickening
- Tumor emboli in dilated dermal lymphatics and vessels
- Diagnosis by punch biopsy
- Mammographic findings may precede clinical findings by several weeks

Post-Operative Breast
- Benign breast biopsy
  - Minimal edema
    - Resolves in one to two months
- Lumpectomy with radiation therapy and axillary dissection
  - Breast firm and fibrotic on clinical breast exam
  - Mammography: Increased density, thickened trabeculae, and thickened skin
  - Improves/resolves two to three years after treatment
  - If findings associated with edema reappear after resolution, suspect recurrence

Breast Edema

Congestive Heart Failure
- Bilateral
  o Most common
- Unilateral
  o Habitual decubitus positioning
- May see pitting edema
  o Absent in non fluid-overload edema
- Mammographic findings resolve with appropriate therapy

Mastitis
- Most commonly occurs in lactating women
  o Affects 1-3% of nursing mothers
- Clinical findings
  o Erythema
  o Warmth
  o Tenderness
  o Possible fever, increased white blood count
- May be complicated by abscess
  o Ultrasound to confirm
- Other causes of breast edema
  o Malignant
    - Locally advanced primary breast cancer
    - Lymphatic obstruction secondary to metastatic nodes
    - Metastatic disease to the breast
    - Lymphoma (secondary)
  o Benign
    - Renal failure
    - Hypoalbuminemia
    - Superior vena cava syndrome

Pathology
- Engorged, dilated lymphatics
- Increased vessel permeability
  o Endothelial damage
- Extracellular water causes spreading of fibers, glands

Clinical Issues
- Important to differentiate benign from malignant causes
  o Thorough history and physical essential

Selected References
1. Oraeuda, CO: Congestive heart failure mimicking inflammatory breast carcinoma: A case report and review of the Literature. Breast Jour 7(2):117-19, 2001
2. Mendelsen, EB: Evaluation of the postoperative breast. Radiologic Clinics of No Amer 30(1):107-38, 1992
3. Doyle, A: Unilateral breast eEdema in congestive heart failure - A mimic of diffuse carcinoma. australus Radial:35:274-75, 1991

Dermal Calcifications

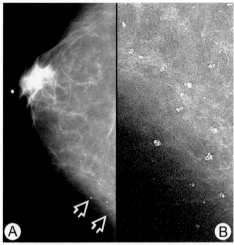

Dermal calcifications. (A) Screening mammogram demonstrates asymptomatic skin calcifications (arrows). The CC mammogram shows their typical medial location. The image magnification view (B) shows the classic appearances of lucent-centered grouped and scattered polygonal and spherical shapes.

Key Facts
- Synonym: Skin calcifications
- Definition: Calcifications within skin sweat glands
- Classic imaging appearance: Lucent-centered grouped or scattered polygonal or spherical calcifications
- Other key facts
  - Sometimes indeterminate
  - Demonstrate on tangential view
  - May require stereotactic localization to confirm dermal location

Imaging Findings
General Features
- Best imaging clue: Multiple, fairly dense, rounded or polygonal calcifications with lucent or umbilicated centers along the edge of breast
- Shape: Rounded, geometric or polygonal
- Size range: 1-2 mm
- Location
  - Most commonly along medial aspect of breast
- Anatomy: Within cutaneous sweat glands
Mammography Findings
- Usually multiple grouped or scattered calcifications
  - Spherical, rounded or polygonal
  - Usually have lucent centers
- Sometimes interrupted, punctate or irregular calcification
  - May require biopsy to confirm
- Localization sometimes necessary
  - Rolled tangential views
  - Stereotactic or grid coordinate localization

Dermal Calcifications

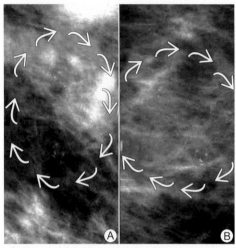

Dermal calcifications. (A) Lateromedial and (B) craniocaudal magnification mammogram showing atypical dermal calcifications. Stereotactic localization established dermal location; core biopsy showed foreign body granulomatous reaction with calcification; etiology unknown.

Ultrasound Findings
- Not helpful

MR Findings
- Not necessary

Imaging Recommendations
- Should suspect on mammography
  - Dismiss when typical or characteristic
  - May require additional workup to confirm
- Specific views
  - Magnification mammography
  - Rolled tangential views
- Skin calcification workup
  - Grid coordinates as with needle localization
  - Skin BB placed over x-y location
  - Orthogonal image with magnification tangential to area covered with BB
- Stereotactic localization
  - Needle tip at skin edge when targeted
- When typical cutaneous location proven, no biopsy required

Differential Diagnosis

Talc in Skin Pores
- Particles more dense, smaller
- No lucent centers
- Very regular distribution

Tattoos
- Pigments may have similar density to calcifications
- Pattern may be evident
- Usually not lucent-centered or polygonal

Dermal Calcifications

Subcutaneous Calcifications
- In subcutaneous fat layer
- May result from prior radiotherapy
- Usually no lucent centers
- Similar prognostic significance

Dermal Foreign Body Giant Cell Reaction
- May have indeterminate calcifications
- Location in skin on tangential views

Skin Scar Calcifications
- Periareolar after reduction mammoplasty
- History prior breast surgery
- Corresponds to known scar

Intramammary Calcifications
- Variable shapes and distributions
- Location within glandular tissue on various views

Pathology
General
- General Path Comments
  o Very common
  o Calcification within sweat glands
  o No clinical significance
- Etiology
  o Physiologic phenomenon
  o May be seen with cystic acne
- Epidemiology
  o Any age, usually > 40

Clinical Issues
Presentation
- Asymptomatic
- Detected at screening mammography
- May be palpable when of significant size

Treatment
- No treatment necessary
- Discuss with patient
  o Advise significance for future reference

Prognosis
- No clinical significance
- No association with malignancy

Selected References
1. Cowie F et al: Subcutaneous calcification as a late effect of orthovoltage chest wall irradiation. Clin Oncol (R Coll Radiol) 11:196-7, 1999
2. Linden SS et al: Breast skin calcifications: Localization with a stereotactic device. Radiology 171:570-1, 1989
3. Berkowitz JE et al: Dermal breast calcifications: Localization with template-guided placement of skin marker. Radiology 163:282, 1987

Diabetic Mastopathy

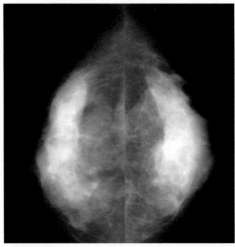

Diabetic mastopathy. CC view of a mammogram of a 50-year-old woman with long-standing insulin-dependent diabetes and stable bilateral firm mass-like breast tissue. (Courtesy E. Siew, MD).

Key Facts
- Synonym: Diabetic fibrous breast disease (DFBD)
- Definition: A variant of fibrosis occurring in diabetics
- Classic imaging appearance
  - Typically obscured by dense breast tissue on mammogram
- Other key facts
  - Present as palpable, firm, nontender masses
  - Usually in premenopausal women
  - Marked sonographic acoustic shadowing
  - Has been reported in diabetic men

Imaging Findings
Mammography Findings
- Surrounding dense parenchyma typically obscures mass(es)
Ultrasound Findings
- Palpable masses show nonspecific findings
- May have marked posterior acoustic shadowing
MR Findings
- T1 C+
  - Focal heterogeneous enhancement
    - Low intensity in early dynamic phase
    - Gradual enhancement over time
    - Heterogeneous spotty on delayed imaging

Differential Diagnosis
Carcinoma
- Suspicious imaging findings lead to biopsy
Focal Fibrosis
- Nonspecific imaging findings of dense parenchyma on mammogram
- Hypoechoic sonographic mass

Diabetic Mastopathy

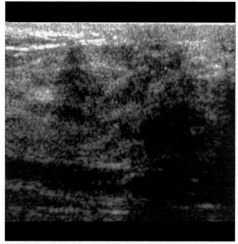

Diabetic mastopathy. Ultrasound of the same case directed to the central firm dense portions of both breasts showed only diffuse shadowing without a focal lesion. (Courtesy E. Siew, MD).

- o Often with posterior acoustic shadowing
- o Often indistinguishable from carcinoma
- o May require biopsy

Other Palpable Nontender Masses With Nonspecific Imaging Findings
- Histologic characterization may be required
  - o Imaging characteristics nonspecific

Pathology
General
- General Path Comments
  - o May be unilateral or bilateral
  - o Lesions are benign
  - o By the time breast symptoms are present patients often have complications of diabetes
    - Retinopathy
    - Nephropathy
    - Neuropathy
- Etiology-Pathogenesis
  - o Findings typically seen in type I insulin-dependent diabetic women
  - o Reported in diabetic men
  - o May be a manifestation of HLA - associated autoimmune disease

Gross Pathologic, Surgical Features
- 2-6 cm in size
- Most not visible as a tumor
- Cut surface often indistinguishable from surrounding breast parenchyma

Microscopic Features
- Collagenous stroma
- Slight increased number of stromal spindle cells
- Prominent myofibroblasts and perivascular lymphocytic infiltrates

Diabetic Mastopathy

Clinical Issues

Presentation
- Mean age of diabetes onset 12, 13 years
- 20 year average interval between diabetes onset and mass
- Premenopausal women
- Palpable, firm, mobile, nontender mass(es)
- Unilateral or bilateral

Natural History
- Self-limited process

Treatment
- Needle core biopsy suggested to establish diagnosis
- Fine needle aspiration (FNA) biopsy may be used to follow patients with recurrent lesions
- Recurrent tumors in a minority of excised cases

Prognosis
- Excellent
- No increased risk for development of invasive cancer

Selected References
1. Rosen PP: Rosen's breast pathology. Lippincott Williams & Wikins, Philadelphia PA; Chapter 3, 53-6, 2001
2. Kopans D: Breast imaging 2nd Edition. Lippincott-Raven, Philadelphia PA; Chapter 19, 562-3, 1998
3. Bassett LW et al: Diagnosis of diseases of the breast. Philadelphia: WB Saunders Co; Chapter 25, 411, 1997

Duct Ectasia

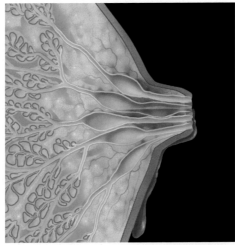

Duct ectasia. Dilated major subareolar ducts are imaged in this drawing. Duct ectasia may be secondary to inflammation, obstruction or glandular atrophy and stasis.

Key Facts
- Synonyms: Mammary duct ectasia, mastitis obliterans
- Definition: Nonspecific subareolar ductal dilatation
- Classic imaging appearance
  - Enlarged tubular retroareolar structures on mammography
- Other key facts
  - Calcifications may be present
  - Fluid or debris-filled, dilated, subareolar ducts on sonography
  - No clinical concern when bilateral and asymptomatic

Imaging Findings
Mammography Findings
- Tubular radiopaque retroareolar structures
- Calcifications may be present
  - Within or around ducts
  - Punctate, coarse rod-like
  - Spherical with lucent centers
Ultrasound Findings
- General features
  - Dilated subareolar ducts coursing to the nipple
  - Internal matrix
    - Anechoic fluid
    - Echogenic debris: May be mobile
MR Findings
- T2WI: Fluid-containing structures are bright
- T1 C+
  - May enhance
  - Intensity less than the normal nipple

Duct Ectasia

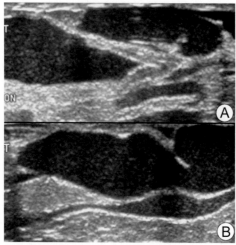

Duct ectasia. Sonogram (A, B) of a 39-year-old nulliparous woman with clinical complaint of chronic galactorrhea while taking the anti-psychotic drug Risperidone shows dilated, fluid-filled, subareolar ducts. Aspiration produced milky fluid.

Imaging Recommendations
- No further imaging following mammography
  - Asymptomatic
  - Multiple
  - No suspicious calcifications
  - No suspicious masses
  - No suspicious distortion

Differential Diagnosis

Ductal Carcinoma In Situ (DCIS)
- Single dilated duct an uncommon presentation of DCIS

Plasma Cell Mastitis
- Benign, rod-like, coarse, linear mammographic calcifications
- Plasmacytic reaction to ductal retained secretion
- May present with a palpable mass

Granulomatous Lobular Mastitis
- No specific pathogenic organism
- Perilobular distribution
- Granulomatous inflammation

Pathology

General
- Dilated major subareolar ducts
  - Occasional involvement of smaller ducts
- Thick or granular secretions
- Etiology-Pathogenesis
  - Not related to parity or breast-feeding
  - May be secondary to
    - Inflammation
    - Obstruction

- Glandular atrophy and stasis
- Epidemiology
  - Tissue atrophy
  - Cigarette smoking
  - Hyperprolactinemia
  - Prolonged phenothiazine exposure

Gross Pathologic, Surgical Features
- Grossly dilated, thick-walled ducts
- Thick or granular secretions

Microscopic Features
- Eosinophilic proteinaceous material
- Foam cells
- Inflammatory changes in ducts and surrounding tissue
- Epithelium may be thin
  - May be replaced by scar

Clinical Issues

Presentation
- Dilated ducts may be palpable
- Nipple discharge
  - Spontaneous
  - Yellow, green or brown

Treatment
- Symptomatic
- Biopsy may be recommended
  - If clinical or imaging characteristics suspicious for carcinoma

Prognosis
- Excellent
- No known associated increased risk for invasive breast cancer

Selected References
1. Rosen PP: Rosen's breast pathology. Lippincott Williams & Wilkins, Philadelphia PA; Chapter 3, 33-9, 2001
2. Bassett LW et al: Diagnosis of diseases of the breast. Philadelphia: WB Saunders Co; Chapter 25, 413-4, 1997
3. Cardenosa G: Breast imaging companion. Lippincott-Raven, Philadelphia PA; 184-7, 1997

Dystrophic Calcifications

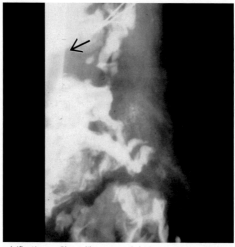

Dystrophic calcifications. Sheet-like coarse & heterogeneous calcifications may be associated within the fibrous capsule surrounding implants. Dystrophic calcifications are present within a fibrous capsule related to a ruptured explanted silicone implant in a woman following reimplantation of a saline implant (arrow).

Key Facts
- Synonyms
  - Heterotopic calcifications
  - Postoperative calcifications
- Definition
  - Benign calcifications typically following breast surgery and radiotherapy
  - More common following addition of radiation therapy
- Classic imaging appearance
  - Large irregular calcifications with lucent centers
- Other key facts
  - May be very extensive
  - Association with silicone breast implants
  - Found in fat necrosis of any cause

Imaging Findings
General Features
- Best imaging clue
  - Large irregular calcifications with lucent centers associated with previous surgery and radiation therapy
- Shape: Irregular, "lava-shaped"
- Size range: > 0.5 mm, typically > 1 mm
- Location - center
  - Adjacent to scar
  - May be subcutaneous
Mammography Findings
- Post-lumpectomy
  - Focal skin tethering and distortion (scarring) with irregular large calcifications
  - May occur up to 4 years after treatment in 30% women

Dystrophic Calcifications

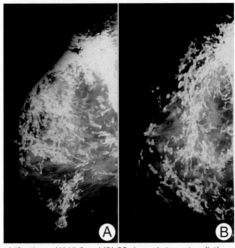

Dystrophic calcifications. (A) MLO and (B) CC views. Late post-radiotherapy extensive bizarre dense dystrophic and heterotopic calcifications, which are largely in the subcutaneous plane.

   o May be intermixed with suspicious calcifications (recurrent malignancy)
- Post-implant
   o Dense irregular calcifications
   o Adjacent to breast implant
   o In fibrotic bed of removed implant
- Post-radiotherapy
   o Usually limited, small numbers of dystrophic calcifications
   o May be very extensive, involving chest wall, subcutaneous tissues

Ultrasound Findings
- Dense echogenic foci associated with hypoechoic scar
- Large calcifications may show posterior shadowing

MR Findings
- No specific findings
- Post-operative scarring and moderate enhancement

Imaging Recommendations
- Dismiss if characteristic
- Correlate with clinical history
- Magnification views for characterization if indeterminate
- Suspicious associated calcifications or focal suspicious mass may require biopsy

Differential Diagnosis

Recurrent Malignancy
- Post-lumpectomy cancer recurrence
- Typically suspicious, small developing calcifications
   o Linear or pleomorphic

Fat Necrosis
- Variable imaging findings
   o Oil cysts
   o Focal stellate mass

Dystrophic Calcifications

Pathology
General
- General Path Comments
  - No specific features
  - Depends on underlying cause
- Etiology-Pathogenesis
  - Nonspecific response to previous insult
  - Post-operative
    - Lumpectomy
    - Post-reduction
    - Post-liposuction
    - Post-implant insertion or removal
  - Post-radiotherapy
  - Post-traumatic (nonsurgical)
- Epidemiology
  - Any age
  - Appropriate prior clinical history

Gross Pathologic, Surgical Features
- No specific findings

Microscopic Features
- Underlying pathology
- Usually some associated fibrosis

Clinical Issues
Presentation
- Screen-detected or on surveillance mammograms
- Prior appropriate clinical history

Treatment
- No specific treatment
- Observation
- Further investigation if suspicious of malignancy

Prognosis
- No malignant potential or associations

Selected References
1. Amin R et al: Subcutaneous calcification following chest wall and breast irradiation: A late complication. Br J Radiol 75:279-82, 2002
2. Bilgen IG et al: Fat necrosis of the breast: Clinical, mammographic and sonographic features. Eur J Radiol 39:92-9, 2001
3. Dershaw DD et al: Patterns of mammographically detected calcifications after breast-conserving therapy associated with tumor recurrence. Cancer 79:1355-61, 1997

Epidermal Inclusion Cyst

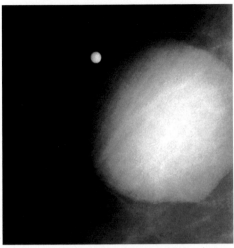

Epidermal inclusion cyst. 78-year-old woman with palpable subcutaneous mass in right axilla. Exaggerated CC view demonstrates a corresponding well-circumscribed, round mass marked as palpable with a BB.

Key Facts
- Definition: Most common epithelial cyst of breast
- Other key facts
  - Arises from skin and adnexa
    - Cutaneous or subcutaneous
  - Often erroneously referred to as sebaceous cyst
    - Imaging and clinical findings indistinguishable
  - No age predilection
  - Reported in males

Imaging Findings
<u>Mammography Findings</u>
- Well-circumscribed mass
  - Portion of border may be ill-defined
- Round
- Isodense to high density
- Superficial
  - Often burned out by appropriate exposure for denser areas
  - Bright light helpful
- Heterogeneous calcifications 20%
- Mammogram may be normal

<u>Ultrasound Findings</u>
- Well-defined, round mass
- Usually hypoechoic
  - Low-level internal echoes
    - Thick intralesional material
- Posterior acoustic enhancement
- Occasionally anechoic or hyperechoic
- Dermal extension evident

Epidermal Inclusion Cyst

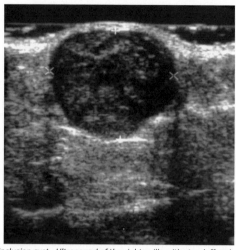

Epidermal inclusion cyst. Ultrasound of the right axilla with standoff pad. Superficial, well-defined hypoechoic mass corresponding to mammographic finding. Note lateral edge refraction, through transmission of sound, and internal echo heterogeneity.

<u>Imaging Recommendations</u>
- Mammography
  - Mark lesion with BB prior to exam
    - Tangential view helpful
    - Demonstrates cutaneous/subcutaneous location
- Ultrasound
  - Standoff pad may be necessary with lower frequency transducers

Differential Diagnosis
<u>Sebaceous Cyst</u>
- Arises from obstructed sebaceous gland
- Contents: Yellow, smooth, buttery material
<u>Fibroadenoma</u>
<u>Cyst</u>
<u>Well-Circumscribed Carcinoma</u>

Pathology
<u>Etiology-Pathogenesis</u>
- Arises from obstructed hair follicle
  - Most common
- May occur along embryonic lines of closure
- Squamous metaplasia of sweat duct
- Traumatic downward implantation of epidermal fragments
  - Reduction mammoplasty
  - FNA or core biopsy
<u>Gross Pathologic, Surgical Features</u>
- Thick contents: White, flaky, waxy
<u>Microscopic Features</u>
- Stratified squamous epithelium

Epidermal Inclusion Cyst

- Nearly identical to epidermis
- Filled with keratin
- Calcifications
- No sebaceous glands

Clinical Issues
Presentation
- Smooth, round, palpable mass
- Movable
- Often visible
- Diagnosis made by needle biopsy
  - Not necessary if characteristic clinical and imaging findings present
- Rupture may lead to inflammatory mass
Treatment
- Controversial
  - Some advocate complete resection
    - Possible malignant potential (extremely rare)
  - Others recommend no intervention
    - Unless inflamed or painful
Prognosis
- Excellent
  - Malignant transformation extremely rare

Selected References
1. Denison, CM: Epidermal inclusion cysts of the breast: Three Lesions with calclifications. Radiology. 204: 493-96, 1997
2. Chantra, PK: Circumscribed fibrocystic mastopathy with formation of epidermal cyst. AJR 163: 831-32, 1994
3. Fajardo LL: Epidermal inclusion cyst after reduction mammoplasty. Radiology 186(1): 103-06, 1993

Extra-Abdominal Desmoid

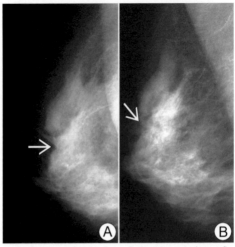

Complaint = enlarging uncomfortable "mass". Erythematous breast firmly attached to chest. Architectural distortion (arrow) only mammographic finding. Core biopsy = DCIS. Intraoperative examination following mastectomy revealed a chest wall mass; Frozen section = benign fibrodysplasia. (Courtesy of Anne Kennedy, MD).

Key Facts
- Synonyms: Fibromatosis, aggressive fibromatosis
- Definition: Aggressive benign proliferation of fibroblasts and collagen
- Classic imaging appearance
  - Spiculated mammographic lesion
- Average size 2.5-3.0 cm
- Extremely rare

Imaging Findings
Mammography Findings
- Irregular spiculated mass
  - No associated calcifications
  - Rarely initially diagnosed by mammography
- Typically close to pectoralis muscle
Ultrasound Findings
- Hypoechoic mass
- Variable posterior acoustic shadowing

Differential Diagnosis
Infiltrative Carcinoma
- Imaging characteristics (spiculated noncalcified mass) indistinguishable from infiltrating carcinoma
Metaplastic Spindle-Cell Carcinoma (Histologic Differential)
- Carcinoma with squamous metaplasia
  - Spectrum of differentiation
  - Mature keratinizing epithelium associated with spindle-cell pseudosarcomatous areas
    - Most of the neoplasm assumes a pseudosarcomatous growth pattern

Extra-Abdominal Desmoid

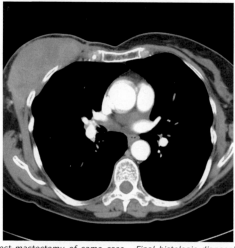

CT scan post-mastectomy of same case. Final histologic diagnosis following mastectomy & chest wall mass biopsy = aggressive fibromatosis. CT scan shows large mass involving (adjacent to) pectoralis. No further treatment has yet been performed & mass continues to grow. (Courtesy of Anne Kennedy, MD).

- Resembles fibromatosis or fibrosarcoma

Trauma
- Reports of direct breast trauma
  - Breast struck by falling concrete
  - Years after drainage of postpartum mastitis

Post-Surgical
- Post breast augmentation

Postoperative Scar
- History key in distinguishing this spiculated lesion from carcinoma

Pathology
General
- General Path Comments
  - Extremely rare, locally aggressive, benign mesenchymal tumor
  - Usually arises in abdominal wall muscle and fascia
  - Size range 1-10 cm
- Epidemiology
  - Association with Gardner's syndrome
    - Familial multiple polyposis
    - Mesenchymal skin tumors
    - Osteomas
    - May have desmoid lesions at mesentery root
  - Association with Familial Multicentric Fibromatosis
  - Reported in association with silicone implants

Gross Pathologic, Surgical Features
- Poorly-circumscribed or ill-defined mass
- Tan, white or gray fibrous tissue

- Cut surface may have whorled appearance

Microscopic Features
- Spindle cells and collagen
- Varied growth patterns in single lesion
- Mitotic figures typically undetectable
- Little cellular pleomorphism

Clinical Issues
Presentation
- Age range 13-80 years
- Palpable firm mass
- May be fixed to pectoralis muscle
- Dimpling or skin retraction may be present

Treatment
- Wide local excision
- Radiation and hormone therapy have been used

Prognosis
- Recurrence rates 21-27%

Selected References
1. Greenburg D et al: Aggressive fibromatosis of the breast: A case report and literature review. The Breast Journal 8:55-7, 2002
2. Rosen PP: Rosen's breast pathology. Lippincott Williams & Wikins, Philadelphia PA; Chapter 40, pp 749-57, 2001
3. Kopans D: Breast imaging 2nd edition. Lippincott-Raven, Philadelphia PA; Chapter 19, pp 563-5, 1998

Fat Necrosis

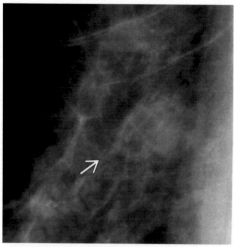

Fat necrosis. 53-year-old woman with non-palpable mass in the lateral right breast, identified on screening mammogram. Cone down CC view right breast shows ill-defined oval mass (arrow) with internal fat. Ultrasound-guided biopsy showed fat necrosis.

Key Facts
- Definition: Benign nonsuppurative process related to breast trauma
- Accidental injury
  - Blunt trauma
    - Direct blow to the thorax
    - Seatbelt injury
  - Penetrating trauma
- Iatrogenic injury
  - Surgery: Biopsy, lumpectomy, transverse rectus abdominis myocutaneous (TRAM) flap, reduction, implant removal
  - Radiation therapy
  - Direct silicone injection
    - Paraffinoma
- No history of prior trauma or surgery 35-50%
- Most common in subareolar and superficial areas near skin
  - More vulnerable to trauma
- Occurs at any age
- Seen in males
- Spontaneous development reported in patients with diabetes or collagen vascular disease
- Imaging findings may be confused with malignancy
  - Biopsy

Imaging Findings
<u>General Features</u>
- Best imaging clue: Oil cyst on mammography
- Size range: Few millimeters to several centimeters
<u>Mammography Findings</u>
- Spiculated area of increased density
  - Fibrosis prominent

Fat Necrosis

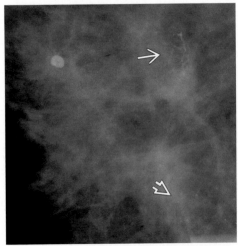

Fat necrosis. 57-year-old women, two years status-post right lumpectomy for DCIS, presented two new areas of calcifications at lumpectomy site. Magnified CC view of surgical site shows the two foci (both biopsy-proven fat necrosis): Superior, lattice-like (arrow) and inferior, punctate calcifications (open arrow).

- o Desmoplastic reaction
- Focal mass
- Band-like density
  - o Seatbelt injury
- Oil cyst
  - o Single or multiple
- Calcifications
  - o Pleomorphic: Branching, rod-like, angular
    - Early manifestation
    - Often evolve to dystrophic or coarse calcifications
    - May be confused with DCIS
  - o Coarse, dystrophic, lucent-centered, eggshell
    - Later manifestation

Ultrasound Findings
- Irregular, hypoechoic mass
  - o Variable enhancement pattern
  - o Corresponding mammographic mass may be spiculated
- Anechoic mass
  - o Well circumscribed
  - o Round to oval
  - o Variable posterior acoustic features
  - o Corresponding oil cyst on mammography
- Complex mass
  - o Mural nodules
  - o Internal bands
  - o May be associated with focal mass or oil cyst on mammography
- Distortion of normal sonographic architecture
  - o Disruption of linear, echogenic fibrotic bands and Cooper's ligaments
  - o Haphazard appearance of fat planes

Fat Necrosis

<u>Imaging Recommendations</u>
- Mammography
- Ultrasound
  - If mammography negative or inconclusive

Differential Diagnosis
<u>Infiltrating Ductal or Lobular Carcinoma</u>
<u>DCIS</u>
<u>Lipoma</u>
<u>Steatocystoma Multiplex</u>
- Bilateral oil cysts
- Not just limited to breast

Pathology
<u>Gross Pathological, Surgical Features</u>
- Firm or hard nodular mass
- Yellowish-white color
- May be associated with recent or old hemorrhage
<u>Microscopic Features</u>
- Loss of nuclei, fusion of adipocytes
  - Damaged cells coalesce
  - Creation of expanded fatty spaces
- Accumulation of foamy histiocytes
  - Fuse into multinucleated giant cells
- Inflammatory reaction: Lymphocytes, polymorphonucleocytes, plasma cells
- Peripheral fibrosis
- Necrotic center

Clinical Issues
<u>Presentation</u>
- May be asymptomatic
  - Discovered on screening mammogram
- Tender, palpable mass or masses
- May be firm, fixed
- Occasionally associated with skin thickening, retraction
- Imaging findings may be preceded by ecchymosis and/or erythema
<u>Treatment</u>
- No treatment usually necessary
- Excision rarely for painful mass
<u>Prognosis</u>
- Excellent
  - No malignant potential

Selected References
1. Kinoshita T, et al. Fat necrosis of breast: A potential pitfall in breast MRI. Clin Imaging 26:250-3, 2002
2. Soo, MS: Fat necrosis in the breast: Sonographic features. Radiology 206:261-96, 1998
3. Hogge, JP et al: The mammographic spectrum of fat necrosis. Radiographics 15:1347-56, 1995

Fibroadenoma

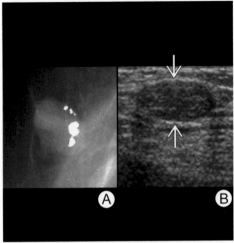

Fibroadenoma. (A) Typical mammographic appearance of an involuting fibroadenoma with eccentric coarse "popcorn" calcifications. (B) Classic sonographic appearance: Oval, well-circumscribed, hypoechoic mass parallel with skin, with slight posterior acoustic enhancement & a thin echogenic rim (arrows).

Key Facts
- Definition: Benign fibroepithelial tumor
  - Most common benign solid mass in women of all ages
- Classic imaging appearance
  - Mammogram – oval well-circumscribed 2 cm mass
  - Sonogram – hypoechoic oval well-circumscribed mass with thin echogenic rim
- May involute following menopause
  - "Popcorn" calcifications

Imaging Findings
Mammography Findings
- Circumscribed mass
  - Oval, lobulated, round
- Low density or isodense to surrounding breast parenchyma
- 1-4 cm in size
- Involuting post-menopausal masses may calcify
  - Begins at periphery and moves toward center
  - May completely replace mass
- May be indistinguishable from cysts
- Atypical appearances
  - May mimic carcinoma
    - Irregular shapes
    - Indistinct or spiculated margins
Ultrasound Findings
- Circumscribed mass
  - Oval
  - Lobulated
  - Round

Fibroadenoma

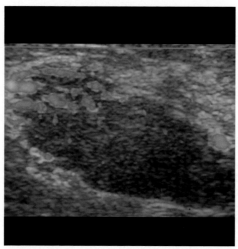

Fibroadenoma. This biopsy-proven fibroadenoma in a premenopausal woman shows prominent vascularity by power Doppler. Unfortunately, the presence or absence of color within a solid breast mass does not reliably distinguish benign from malignant lesions.

- Homogeneous, low-level, internal echogenicity
  - May have heterogeneous internal echogenicity
- Often with thin echogenic rim
- Posterior acoustic enhancement may be prominent
- Atypical appearances
  - May mimic carcinoma
    - Irregular or microlobulated margins
    - Posterior acoustic shadowing

MR Findings
- Large lesions may be bright on T2WI
- Typically oval
- Smooth or lobulated borders
- Variable enhancement patterns based on histologic components
  - Strong contrast uptake
    - Adenomatous and myxoid lesions
  - No or delayed enhancement
    - Fibrous lesions
- May have nonenhancing internal septations
- Limited in differentiating equivocal mammographic or sonographic lesions

Imaging Recommendations
- If < 30 years begin work up with ultrasound
  - Imaging and clinical surveillance may be appropriate
- If > 30 years mammography and ultrasound for appropriate work up
- Clinical and imaging characteristics determine biopsy recommendations

Differential Diagnosis
Tubular Adenoma
- Uncommon
- Dominant tubular elements with minimal stroma

Fibroadenoma

Lactating Adenoma
- Pregnant and lactating women
- Prominent tubular and lobular elements with secretory activity

Phyllodes
- Older patients
- Larger lesions
- Cystic spaces within otherwise sonographically similar lesions
- Histologic differences

Pathology
General
- General Path Comments
  - Benign tumor with varying amounts of epithelial and fibrous elements
  - 1/5 of all breast masses
  - Multiple tumors in 15%
  - 10% breast masses in post menopausal women

Gross Pathologic, Surgical Features
- Firm rubbery circumscribed mass
- Clear identification from surrounding tissue
- No true capsule

Microscopic Features
- Proliferation of glandular and stromal elements
- Two growth patterns
  - Intracanalicular
  - Pericanalicular
  - No prognostic difference
- More proliferative epithelium and more cellular stroma
  - < 20-year-old women
- Less cellular stroma, hyalinization and fibrosis
  - Postmenopausal
  - May calcify

Clinical Issues
Presentation
- Painless, firm mass
- Mean age = 30
- May be image detected

Treatment
- Clinical and sonographic follow-up may be appropriate
- Palpable masses may warrant tissue sampling
  - Then followed clinically and with imaging
- Biopsy recommended for atypical findings
- Any growing mass in postmenopausal woman warrants biopsy consideration despite prior diagnosis

Prognosis
- Excellent
- Risk of carcinoma within lesion = general population risk

Selected References
1. Rosen PP: Breast pathology diagnosis by needle core biopsy. Lippincott Williams & Wikins, Philadelphia PA. Chapter 7, 65-70, 1999
2. Friedrich M: MRI of the breast: State of the art. Eur Radiol 8:707-25, 1998
3. Bassett LW et al: Diagnosis of diseases of the breast. Philadelphia: WB Saunders Co. Chapter 25, 385-94, 1997

Fibroadenolipoma

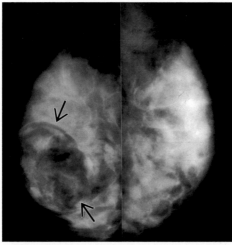

Fibroadenolipoma. 44-year-old with stable palpable mass (indicated on the mammogram). Characteristics are those of well-encapsulated, fat-containing mass or "breast-within-a-breast" appearance.

Key Facts
- Synonyms: Hamartoma, fibroadenolipoma, lipofibroadenoma, adenolipofibroma,
- Definition: Encapsulated fat and glandular element proliferation
- Classic imaging appearance
  - "Breast-within-a-breast" well-encapsulated mammographic mass
- Other key facts
  - Typically a mammographic finding
  - Benign
  - Uncommon

Imaging Findings
Mammography Findings
- If pseudocapsule can be seen, these are round or oval well-circumscribed lesions
- Varying mixtures of fat and fibroglandular tissue elements
Ultrasound Findings
- Well-circumscribed
- Pseudocapsule may reflect echoes
- Mixture of sonolucent (fat) and heterogeneous echogenic patterns
Imaging Recommendations
- No further imaging recommendations when typical mammographic pattern is present

Differential Diagnosis: Fat-Containing Well-Encapsulated Lesions
Galactoceles
- Most are radiolucent, smoothly margined masses
- Lesions contain fat and inspissated secretions
- May demonstrate a fat-fluid level on lateral mammogram

Fibroadenolipoma

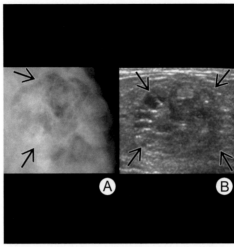

Fibroadenolipoma. Lactating woman with stable right breast mass unaffected by hormonal stimulation of pregnancy or lactation. Mammogram shows encapsulated fat-containing mass. Ultrasound shows a mixture of low-level and heterogeneous echoes surrounded by a pseudocapsule (arrows).

Hibernoma
- Located in axillary tail or axilla
- Contain brown fat

Fibrolipoma
- Mature adipose tissue and collagenous stroma
- Slightly prominent fibroblasts

Chondrolipoma
- Mature adipose tissue and hyaline cartilage
- No calcifications on mammography
- Benign; have been treated with excisional biopsy

Oil Cysts
- Small, round, internally lucent masses with calcified rims

Fibroadenoma
- Lesion may be suspected as a fibroadenoma
  - If capsule is not clearly defined (or detected) on mammogram
  - When little fat is present

Pathology

General
- Hamartoma definition
  - A focal malformation that resembles a neoplasm, but results from faulty development in an organ
  - It is composed of an abnormal mixture of tissue elements, or an abnormal proportion of a single element normally present at that site
- Adenolipoma is most common variant of mammary hamartoma
- Size range up to 13 cm
- Reports of misclassifcation of cases of pseudoangiomatous stromal hyperplasia (PASH) as hamartomas

Fibroadenolipoma

Gross Pathologic, Surgical Features
- Cut surface has a variegated mix of fat and fibrous parenchyma
  o Surrounded by a thin fibrous pseudocapsule
- Cysts may be present

Microscopic Features
- Fat mixed in varying proportions with mammary parenchyma
- Pseudocapsule = compressed breast tissue
- Lobules & ducts appear normal
- Little or no proliferative change
- Lacks adenomatous component in fibroadenomas with adipose metaplasia
- No cytologic atypia as seen in phyllodes tumors with adipose stroma

Clinical Issues

Presentation
- Typically a mammographic finding
- When palpable, mass is painless
- Reported to cause breast enlargement without any frank mass
- Age range 20-80 years
- Mean age of 45 years

Treatment
- No treatment necessary unless appearance is atypical

Prognosis
- Excellent

Selected References
1. Rosen PP: Rosen's breast pathology. Lippincott Williams & Wikins, Philadelphia PA; Chapter 40, 779-81, 2001
2. Altermatt HJ et al: Multiple hamartomas of the breast. Appl Pathol 7:145-8, 1989
3. Stedman's medical dictionary, 24th ed. Baltimore; Williams & Wilkins 619, 1982

Focal Fibrosis

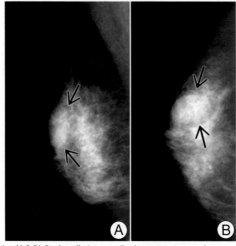

Focal fibrosis. (A & B) Oval, well-circumscribed, upper outer quadrant mammographic mass (arrows). Ultrasound-guided biopsy showed focal fibrosis and fibrocystic change.

Key Facts
- Synonyms: Focal fibrosis of the breast, breast sclerosis, fibrous mastopathy
- Definition: Benign stromal proliferation
- Classic imaging appearance: Noncalcified mass on mammography and sonography
- Other key facts
  - Incidence in resected specimens 2-8%
  - Benign

Imaging Findings
Mammography Findings
- Mass
  - Shape
    - Oval
    - Round
    - Lobulated
  - Margins
    - Obscured
    - Circumscribed
    - Ill-defined
- Asymmetric density
- Architectural distortion
Ultrasound Findings
- Mass
  - Shape
    - Oval
    - Irregular
  - Margins
    - Well-circumscribed

Focal Fibrosis

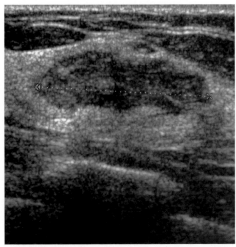

Focal fibrosis. Ultrasound of the same case shows a lobulated, fairly well-circumscribed, hypoechoic lesion parallel to the skin with no posterior acoustic effect. Ultrasound-guided biopsy showed focal fibrosis and fibrocystic change.

- Ill-defined
  - o Internal echogenicity
    - Hypoechoic with central "cloud-like" echogenicity
    - Isoechoic
    - Heterogeneous
  - o Posterior acoustic features
    - No effect
    - Posterior acoustic shadowing
    - Posterior acoustic enhancement
- Acoustic shadowing without mass

Imaging Recommendations
- Mammography and ultrasound
- Reported findings with core biopsy
  - o 9% of core biopsies
  - o Mammographic findings
    - Mass
    - Density
    - Microcalcifications
  - o Sonographic findings
    - Hypoechoic mass
    - Oval or irregular
    - Most without posterior enhancement or shadowing
  - o Careful radiology-pathology correlation
  - o Imaging follow-up may be advised

Differential Diagnosis

Carcinoma
- Imaging characteristics include many of those reported for focal fibrosis
- Biopsy recommended when imaging characteristics are suspicious

Focal Fibrosis

Fibroadenoma
- Similar imaging characteristics on both mammogram and ultrasound

Pathology
General
- General Path Comments
  - Focal areas of fibrous tissue
  - Obliteration of acini and ducts
- Etiology-Pathogenesis
  - Hormonal stimulation specific to fibroelastic tissue
    - Predominantly pre-menopausal women
  - Normal variant of involution
  - End result of inflammatory process
Microscopic Features
- Perilobular
  - Perilobular stroma elastic fibers displaced by dense collagen
  - Collagen rings may form small nodule
  - Ducts and acini may be obliterated
- Septal fibrosis
  - Dense collagenous bands run between adipose lobules
  - May expand to form mass-like lesion
- Haphazard fibrosis
  - Involves interlobular stroma
  - Thick collagen fibers radiate from a central focus
  - May contract to form a scar

Clinical Issues
Presentation
- May be palpable
  - Usually painless
  - Painful mass
    - Uncommon
- Usually an imaging finding
Treatment
- Based on clinical and imaging level of suspicion
- Findings at core biopsy may be sufficient
  - Must have radiologic/pathologic concordance
  - Excisional biopsy may be necessary
Prognosis
- Excellent

Selected References
1. Revelon G et al: Focal fibrosis of the breast: Imaging characteristics and histopathologic correlation. Radiology 216:255-9, 2000
2. Rosen EL et al: Focalfibrosis: A common breast lesion diagnosed at imaging-guided core biopsy. AJR 173:1657-62, 1999
3. Venta LA et al: Imaging features of focal breast fibrosis: Mammographic-pathologic correlation of noncalcified breast lesions. AJR 173:309-16, 1999

Galactocele

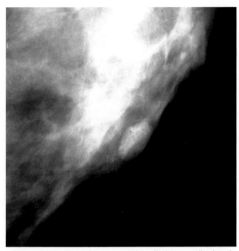

Galactocele. Spot mammogram shows an oval, well-circumscribed, palpable mass in a 38-year-old lactating woman. Fine needle aspiration was inconclusive and sonogram demonstrated shadowing. Excisional biopsy revealed a galactocele and lactational breast tissue changes.

Key Facts
- Definition: Benign lesion that contains milk-like-fluid
- Classic imaging appearance: Well-circumscribed mass
- Other key facts
  - Cysts contain fat and inspissated secretions
  - Most occur in pregnant or lactating women
  - Reported in female and male infants
  - May be seen with chronic galactorrhea
    - Pituitary adenoma
    - Prolactin-stimulating pharmaceuticals

Imaging Findings
Mammography Findings
- Fat-containing, well-circumscribed mass
  - May be indistinguishable from other well-circumscribed masses
  - May demonstrate fat-fluid levels on lateral projection
  - May be associated with fat necrosis
- Mottled appearance similar to hamartoma has been described
  - Likened to curdled milk
Ultrasound Findings
- Well-circumscribed mass often with thin echogenic rim
  - Low-level internal echoes
  - May have posterior acoustic enhancement
  - Focal echogenic areas and distal shadowing may be seen
  - Findings often nonspecific
  - Correlate with mammogram and history

Differential Diagnosis
Simple Cyst
- May be indistinguishable on mammogram

Galactocele

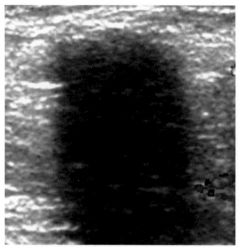

Galacotcele. Ultrasound of the same mass demonstrates a suspicious mass with indistinct margins, marked hypoechogenicity & posterior acoustic shadowing. Biopsy findings (galactocele & lactational changes) found no direct histologic correlate to explain the prominent posterior acoustic shadowing.

- Ultrasound should be definitive for diagnosis

Complex Cyst
- Mass on mammogram
- Ultrasound may be helpful
- Aspiration often required

Fat-Containing Well-Circumscribed Masses
- Encapsulated fat-containing masses are benign
- Do not require further diagnostic imaging or intervention

Pathology

General
- General Path Comments
  - Benign
  - Solitary or multiple well-circumscribed unilateral or bilateral masses
  - Average size = 2 cm
  - Lesions > 5 cm reported
- Etiology-Pathogenesis
  - Secondary to ductal dilatation

Gross Pathologic, Surgical Features
- Masses
- Milk-like fluid and inspissated secretions

Microscopic Features
- Epithelial lined cysts
- Cytoplasmic vacuolization secondary to lipid
- Apocrine metaplasia may be present
- Intact cysts
  - Surrounded by fibrous material without inflammation
- Ruptured cysts
  - Chronic inflammatory response

o Possible fat necrosis

Clinical Issues
<u>Presentation</u>
- Palpable mass
  - o Pregnant
  - o Lactating
  - o Early post-lactational setting
  - o Stimulated by hyperprolactinemic state
    - ▪ Pituitary adenoma
    - ▪ Pharmaceuticals

<u>Treatment</u>
- Aspiration typically treatment of choice
- Questionable cases may require surgical excision
- Milk fistula a rare complication of incomplete surgical excision

<u>Prognosis</u>
- Excellent

Selected References
1. Sawhney S et al: Sonographic appearances of galactoceles. J Clin Ultrasound 30:18-22, 2002
2. Rosen PP: Rosen's breast pathology. Lippincott Williams & Wikins, Philadelphia PA; chapter 3, 32-3, 2001
3. Kopans D: Breast imaging 2nd edition. Lippincott-Raven, Philadelphia PA; chapter 19, 557-8, 1998

Glandular Islands

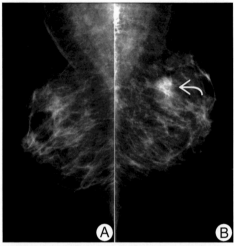

Glandular islands. (A & B) MLO projections from a 4-view screening mammogram show a prominent asymmetric density in left upper outer quadrant (curved arrow). Patient was recalled for further workup views. Proven glandular island.

Key Facts
- Synonyms
  - Focal asymmetric glandular tissue
  - Asymmetric density
- Definition
  - Focal area of glandular tissue separate from main glandular cone
- Classic imaging appearance
  - Asymmetric, focal, rounded, soft-tissue, low-density area with mottled, internal, fatty density
- Other key facts
  - May mimic true mass on mammography
  - May become more conspicuous with surrounding tissue atrophy

Imaging Findings
General Features
- Best imaging clue
  - No frank mass-like characteristics
  - Internal fatty density helpful for diagnosis
- Shape
  - Usually convex contour
  - May have rounded contour
- Size range
  - 1-5 cm diameter
- Location
  - Along edge of breast cone
  - Not retroareolar region
  - Usually upper outer quadrant
Mammography Findings
- Focal area separate from glandular tissue
- Homogeneous or mixed internal density

Glandular Islands

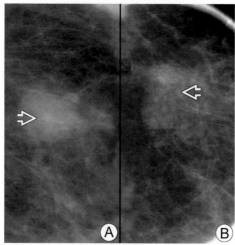

Glandular islands. Coned magnification (A) MLO and (B) CC views in the same patient show a focal asymmetric density (arrows) that contains a mixture of soft tissue and fatty densities typical of glandular tissue. Negative ultrasound, no palpable lump. Biopsy-proven glandular tissue .

- Usually spreads on compression views

Ultrasound Findings
- Identical to normal parenchyma

MR Findings
- All sequences
  - Identical to normal parenchyma

Imaging Recommendations
- Mammography usually diagnostic
- Probably glandular tissue when
  - Mammographically persistent focal density
  - Negative detailed ultrasound
  - No palpable lesion
- Rarely requires biopsy confirmation
- Ultrasound useful to exclude focal lesion
- Short-term follow-up rarely required

Differential Diagnosis

Pseudoangiomatous Stromal Hyperplasia (PASH)
- Common in developing asymmetric densities
- Benign proliferation of fibrosis
- Contains slit-like pseudovascular spaces
- Electron microscopy: Spaces acellular or lined by fibroblasts

Fibroadenolipoma
- Breast hamartoma
- Fat–containing encapsulated lesion
- Contains fat and glandular density
- Usually within or in contact with glandular cone

Glandular Islands

Pathology

<u>General</u>
- General Path Comments
  - Rarely biopsied
- Etiology-Pathogenesis
  - Normal variation
  - Related to combination hormone replacement therapy (HRT)
    - May "appear" while on HRT
    - Resolves on cessation
    - Less common with estrogen only HRT
- Epidemiology
  - Usually > 40
  - Often postmenopausal

<u>Gross Pathologic, Surgical Features</u>
- No focal mass

<u>Microscopic Features</u>
- Normal parenchymal ductal and lobular elements

Clinical Issues

<u>Presentation</u>
- Asymptomatic
- If palpable, further evaluation is mandatory
- Usually screen detected
- Increased frequency on combination HRT

<u>Natural History</u>
- Stable or reduces over time
- With combination estrogen/progestin HRT
  - May coalesce with other islands
    - Forms larger glandular areas
    - Resolves on cessation of HRT

<u>Treatment</u>
- Reassurance, return to routine surveillance
- Regular clinical or breast self-examination
- Short-term follow-up imaging rarely useful
- Needle biopsy confirmation rarely needed

<u>Prognosis</u>
- No prognostic significance

Selected References
1. Lee CH et al: Follow-up of breast lesions diagnosed as benign with stereotactic core-needle biopsy: Fequency of mammographic change and false-negative rate. Radiology 212:189-94, 1999
2. Piccoli CW et al: Developing asymmetric breast tissue. Radiology 211:111-7, 1999
3. Dawson JS et al: Short-term recall for 'probably benign' mammographic lesions detected in a three yearly screening programme. Clin Radiol 49:391-5, 1994

Granulomatous Mastitis

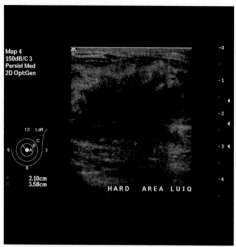

Granulomatous mastitis. Ultrasound in six-month postpartum woman with a hard, indurated breast, clinical signs of inflammation & sinuses draining pus from the skin shows a focal, irregular, markedly, hypoechoic mass with increased surrounding echogenicity (edema) most consistent in this setting with an inflammatory mass.

Key Facts
- Synonyms: Idiopathic mastitis, nonspecific mastitis, granulomatous lobular mastitis, nonspecific granulomatous mastitis
- Definition: Noninfective granulomatous inflammation of the breast
- Imaging appearance
  - Focal dense area on mammography
  - Irregular, clustered, hypoechoic regions on ultrasound
  - Nonspecific appearance with wide differential
- Other key facts
  - Probably autoimmune etiology
  - Often postpartum: Breast-feeding history
  - Inflammatory mass with discharging sinuses

Imaging Findings
General Features
- Best imaging clue: Irregular hypoechoic regions on ultrasound
Mammography Findings
- Focal, poorly-defined increased parenchymal density
Ultrasound Findings
- Multiple clustered, often contiguous, tubular hypoechoic lesions
- Large irregular hypoechoic mass(es)
- Hypoechoic linear tracks to skin (cutaneous sinuses)
MR Findings
- T2WI
  - Microabscesses – small pockets of hyperintense pus
- T1 C+
  - Intensely enhancing region(s)
  - Markedly irregular boundaries
  - Nonenhancing focal areas (containing pus)

Granulomatous Mastitis

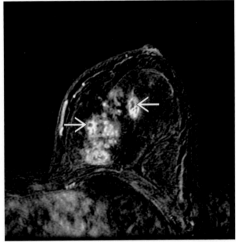

Granulomatous mastitis. Contrast-enhanced MRI in the same woman, showing multiple adjacent areas of intensely enhancing inflammatory tissue surrounding small, nonenhancing pockets of pus (arrows). MRI depicts the extent of the inflammation better than ultrasound, mammography or clinical examination.

Differential Diagnosis
Diffuse or Inflammatory Breast Carcinoma
- No discharging sinuses or pus
- Needle biopsy usually confirms

Bacterial Mastitis
- Culture required to differentiate
- Draining sinuses uncommon

Other Infective Nonbacterial Mastitis
- Culture usually required for diagnosis
- Potential organisms
  o Tuberculosis
  o Mycobacterium abscesses
  o Fungal infection (e.g., sparganosis)
  o Actinomycosis
  o Histoplasmosis
  o Brucellosis

Other Systemic Granulomatous Conditions
- Non-puerperal
- Breast findings rarely first presentation of condition
- Wegener's granulomatosis
- Sarcoidosis

Cholesterol Granulomas of the Breast
- Foreign body reaction
- No discharging pus
- Diagnosis usually made incidentally

Oil Granulomas
- Always history of cosmetic enhancement
- Paraffin oil injections
  o May be apparent only on biopsy

Granulomatous Mastitis

- Silicone oil granulomas
  - History of prior silicone breast implants
  - History of breast injections (Asia)
  - Radiographically dense droplets

Pathology
General
- Etiology
  - Probably autoimmune
  - Triggering incident lactation; sometimes spontaneous
- Epidemiology
  - Parous women
  - Typically postpartum

Gross Pathologic, Surgical Features
- Irregular area of poorly-defined inflammation
- Thick pus in multiple microabscesses

Microscopic Features
- Cytology suggestive
- Histology characteristic
  - Noncaseating granulomas
  - Epithelioid cells
  - Multinucleated Langhans-type giant cells
  - Neutrophils, lymphocytes, and stromal cells
  - No acid-fast bacilli, fungi, oil or cholesterol deposits
  - No organisms on culture

Clinical Issues
Presentation
- Usually postpartum, breast-feeding almost universal
  - May have erythema nodosum (rare)
- Clinical signs of inflammation
  - Tenderness and mass
  - Skin reddening & warmth
  - Pus discharging from skin sinuses & nipple

Natural History
- May resolve spontaneously
- Often relapses intermittently
- May recur metachronously in opposite breast

Treatment
- Oral steroid therapy usually resolves completely
- Surgical excision usually not successful
- Antibiotic and antituberculous therapy limited benefit

Prognosis
- Excellent if treated correctly

Selected References
1. Sakurai T et al: A case of granulomatous mastitis mimicking breast carcinoma. Breast Cancer 9:265-8, 2002
2. Yilmaz E et al: Mammographic and sonographic findings in the diagnosis of idiopathic granulomatous mastitis. Eur Radiol 11:2236, 2001
3. Martinez-Parra D et al: Utility of fine-needle aspiration in the diagnosis of granulomatous lesions of the breast. Diagn Cytopathol 17:108, 1997

Hemangioma

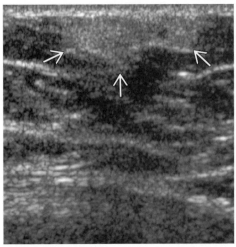

Ultrasound of subcutaneous hemangioma. Lesion presented as mammographically detected asymmetric density, shown to be subcutaneous on workup views and ultrasound (arrows). Biopsy proven.

Key Facts
- Synonyms
  - Cavernous hemangioma
  - Perilobular hemangioma
  - Subcutaneous hemangioma
- Definition
  - Benign well-circumscribed vascular neoplasm
  - Tangled small normal vessels
- Classic imaging appearance
  - Hyperechoic mass on ultrasound
  - Markedly hyperintense mass on T2W MRI
- Almost always slow-flow lesions
- Most occur in adult women
- May rarely occur in female children and men
- Histological atypia may occur
  - No progression to angiosarcoma documented
  - Biopsy to exclude malignancy

Imaging Findings
General Features
- Best imaging clues
  - Hyperechoic compressible mass on US
  - Increased flow on power Doppler
- Other features
  - Shape: Lobulated with indistinct margins
  - Size range: Few mm to 2 cm
  - > 2 cm: Must exclude angiosarcoma
- Subcutaneous lesions show bluish skin discoloration
Mammography Findings
- Poorly-defined soft-tissue density/mass

Hemangioma

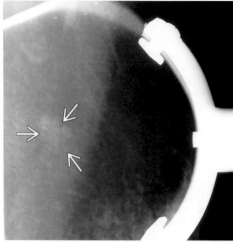

Mammogram of the same case. The patient was recalled for assessment after screening mammography for this indeterminate nodule in the upper outer quadrant. Spot compression mammogram shows an indistinct, lobulated, soft-tissue nodule with no calcifications (arrows).

- No characteristic findings
- Calcifications & phleboliths unusual

Ultrasound Findings
- General
  - Hyperechoic mass
  - Indistinct margins typical
  - Can be partially compressed
- Flow findings
  - Increased flow on color or power Doppler study
  - Enhance with US contrast agents

MR Findings
- T1: No specific features
- T2WI: Markedly hyperintense mass
- Other sequences – slow intense gadolinium enhancement

Differential Diagnosis

Hyperechoic Breast Carcinoma
- Uncommon ultrasound appearance
- Typically infiltrating ductal carcinoma
- Non-compressible

Angiosarcoma
- Malignant primary vascular tumor
- Often very large
- Low-grade lesions difficult to distinguish

Angiomatosis
- Diffuse mass-like lesion
- Mixture of hemangiomatous & lymphangiomatous channels

Kasabach-Merritt Syndrome
- Multiple systemic hemangiomas, may be malignant

Hemangioma

- Aka Hemangioma with thrombocytopenia
- Thrombocytopenia with coagulopathy
- Highly hypervascular high flow mass(es)

Pathology
General
- Capillary, cavernous or venous subtypes
- Perilobular found incidentally
- Etiology-Pathogenesis
  - Unknown
  - May be developmental in neonates
- Epidemiology
  - Mostly women > 25 yo
  - Rarely female infants and children
  - Extremely rare in men

Gross Pathologic, Surgical Features
- Typically well-defined mass
- 50% have non-neoplastic "feeding vessel"

Microscopic Features
- Cavernous or capillary
  - Thin-walled, blood-filled vascular spaces
  - Separated by fibrous septa
  - Extensive fibrosis
  - Sometimes phleboliths
- Venous
  - Circumscribed disorderly vascular proliferation
  - Mainly venous channels

Clinical Issues
Presentation
- Soft-tissue mass on screening mammogram or US
- Palpable mass or thickening

Natural History
- Children: May spontaneously resolve
- Adults: No progression in most cases

Treatment
- Core needle biopsy recommended
- No treatment if benign, typical
- Excision if atypia to exclude angiosarcoma

Prognosis
- Excellent

Selected References
1. Siewert B et al: Sonographic evaluation of subcutaneous hemangioma of the breast. AJR 178:1025-7, 2002
2. Hoda SA et al: Hemangiomas of the breast with atypical histological features. Further analysis of histological subtypes confirming their benign character. Am J Surg Pathol 16:553-60, 1992
3. Jozefczyk MA: Vascular tumors of the breast. II. Perilobular hemangiomas and hemangiomas. Am J Surg Pathol 9:491-503, 1985

Hematoma

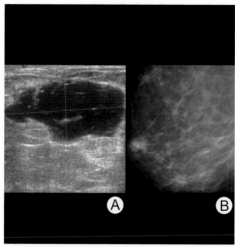

Hematoma. 61-year-old woman following core biopsy and clip placement. (A) Shows a large hematoma (day 10 following the core biopsy) and the needle localization was postponed. (B) Is the mammogram 7 weeks after the core. The residual hematoma can be seen as a soft tissue mass around the clip.

Key Facts
- Definition: Localized mass of extravasated blood within breast
- Occupies either a surgical cavity or traumatic tear
  - May spread into parenchyma, connective tissue, or adipose tissue
- Most common problem resulting from trauma to breast
- Should resolve spontaneously without intervention
- Clinical history important for diagnosis
  - Imaging findings often mimic malignancy

Imaging Findings
<u>Mammography Findings</u>
- Early changes
  - Round or oval mass
  - Margins variable
    - Ill-defined
    - Sharp
    - Better defined as hematoma organizes
  - Air-fluid levels occasionally observed in post-op collections
  - Diffuse density
    - Interstitial spread
  - Skin thickening
- Late changes
  - Decrease in size over time
  - Persistent residual skin thickening
    - Usually completely resolves
  - Spiculated mass
  - Architectural distortion
  - Fat necrosis
- Seatbelt injury

Hematoma

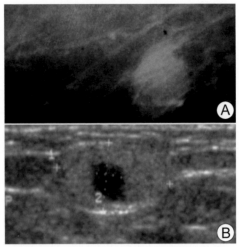

Hematoma. Palpable mass in the medial right breast following a seatbelt injury. Spot mag (A) demonstrates an oval, superficial, smooth, dense, mass with partially obscured margins. US (B) = oval, smooth, complex cystic mass with a focal, markedly hypolucent center. Findings resolved 6 weeks.

  o Band-like density

Ultrasound Findings
- Early changes
  o Ill-defined mass
    ▪ Variable acoustic enhancement
  o Architectural distortion
- Late changes
  o More sharply demarcated with time
  o Usually hypoechoic
  o Echogenic internal components
    ▪ Fluctuant with palpation
    ▪ Distinguished from solid lesion

MR Findings
- T1 C-
  o Variable signal intensity
    ▪ Age related
- T1 C+
  o Minimal to moderate enhancement
  o Somewhat delayed enhancement

Imaging Recommendations
- Not required if diagnosis is clinically obvious
- Mammography
  o Wait at least two weeks after aspiration or biopsy
    ▪ Mammographic opacity may obscure significant breast pathology
    ▪ Reduces false positives
- Ultrasound as adjunct to mammography

Hematoma

Differential Diagnosis
Contusion
- Subtle diffuse infiltration of tissues by blood or edema
  - Blood dissects along tissue planes
- Mammography
  - Mild architectural distortion and trabecular thickening
  - Rarely produces mass
Cyst
Seroma
- Cannot distinguish from hematoma on mammography or ultrasound
- Occupies post-op cavity
Carcinoma
- Meticulous history essential

Pathology
General
- Etiology
  - Iatrogenic
    - Surgery: Lumpectomy, excisional biopsy, augmentation, reduction
    - Core biopsy
    - FNA or cyst aspiration
  - Non-iatrogenic
    - Trauma
  - Arterial disruption
    - Medial breast
    - Internal mammary artery
    - Perforators through chest wall
    - Lateral breast, axillary artery
    - Lateral thoracic branch

Clinical Issues
Presentation
- Painful, palpable mass after known trauma or surgery
  - Occasionally occurs spontaneously
    - Anticoagulant therapy
    - Underlying carcinoma
- Ecchymosis, skin discoloration
- Cannot distinguish from post-op seroma clinically
- Clinical symptoms usually completely resolve
  - Post-traumatic: Up to six weeks
  - Post-lumpectomy: Up to one year
Treatment
- Small
  - Supportive care: Ice pack (acute), warm compresses, analgesia
- Large, painful
  - Aspiration or surgical drainage

Selected References
1. Myhre, A et al: Hemorrhage into the breast in a restrained driver after a motor vehicle collision. AJR 179:690, 2002
2. Nagasawa, M et al: Sudden hemorrhage of the breast caused by breast cancer: A Case Report and Review of the Literature. Breast Cancer. 7(2):176-8, 2000
3. Mendelson EB. Evaluation of the postoperative breast. Radiol Clin North Am 30:107-38, 1992

Hyperplasia, Usual Ductal

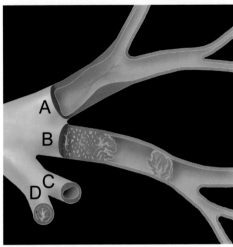

Various types of ductal hyperplasia. (A) Mild hyperplasia. (B) Moderate hyperplasia with epithelial bridging. (C) Florid hyperplasia, streaming pattern. (D) Florid hyperplasia, fenestrated pattern.

Key Facts
- Synonyms: Ductal intraepithelial neoplasia (DIN) 1a, ordinary ductal hyperplasia, epitheliosis, papillomatosis
- Definition: Proliferative increased cellularity of glandular ductal epithelium beyond two layers, without cellular atypia or malignant features
- No classic imaging appearance
- Part of spectrum of DIN (DIN 1abc, 2, 3)
  - IDH ("usual" intraductal hyperplasia, DIN 1a)
  - ADH (atypical intraductal hyperplasia, DIN 1b/1c)
  - DCIS (ductal carcinoma in situ, DIN 1c/2/3)
- Other key facts
  - Physiological in pregnancy
  - Form of benign proliferative breast disease (BPPD)
  - Variable pathologic diagnostic agreement
  - Modest increased risk for subsequent breast carcinoma

Imaging Findings
General
- No specific imaging features
Mammography Findings
- Asymmetric or nonspecific density
- Parenchymal distortion
- Indeterminate microcalcifications
Ultrasound Findings
- Focal thickening of glandular parenchyma
- Associated focal lesion (e.g., papilloma, radial scar, cyst)
MR Findings
- No specific findings; usually identical to normal parenchyma
Imaging Recommendations
- No imaging test useful for diagnosis

Hyperplasia, Usual Ductal

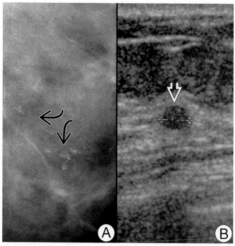

(A) CC magnification shows indeterminate clustered microcalcifications (curved arrows). Core biopsy: Benign calcifications and IDH. (B) US of palpable lesion: Hypoechoic, rounded, nonspecific nodule (open arrow). Excisional biopsy showed usual ductal hyperplasia mixed with sclerosing and blunt duct adenosis.

Differential Diagnosis
Juvenile Papillomatosis
- Adolescents and young women
- Papillary neoplasms with connecting papillary ductal proliferation
- Sometimes classified as variant of IDH

Adenosis, Blunt Duct Adenosis
- Proliferation of epithelial & myoepithelial cells in terminal ductal lobular unit (TDLU)
- Well-defined nodule (nodular adenosis), poorly-defined lesion (tubular, sclerosing), or clustered microcalcifications (sclerosing adenosis)

Fibrocystic Changes
- Gross or microscopic cysts, apocrine hyperplasia, mild epithelial hyperplasia and mild adenosis
- May have indeterminate microcalcifications

Atypical Ductal Hyperplasia
- Variant of florid ductal hyperplasia with cellular atypia or malignancy
- Confined distribution, does not meet criteria for DCIS
- Often indeterminate microcalcifications

Ductal Carcinoma In Situ, Low Grade
- Intraductal proliferation of malignant cells
- Indeterminate or malignant microcalcifications on screening mammogram

Pathology
General
- Any increase in cellularity from normal
- No cellular atypia or malignancy
- New DIN classification emphasizes spectrum of changes
- Continuum concept (IDH→ADH→DCIS) challenged by molecular pathology
- Wide range of disagreement about levels of hyperplasia & atypia
- Pathogenesis: Unknown; from cytokeratin-5 (Ck-5)-positive stem cells

Hyperplasia, Usual Ductal

- Epidemiology
  - Women, any age (usually 30-60), especially on hormone replacement therapy (HRT); median 45
  - Men with gynecomastia
  - Up to 30% of benign biopsies

Gross Pathologic, Surgical Features
- No specific findings; may have firm area of tissue

Microscopic Features
- Isolated, segmental or multicentric
- Pure epithelial or mixed epithelial, myoepithelial and apocrine cells
- Various growth patterns
  - Micropapillary: Irregular fronds, often short
  - "Streaming" or spindling: Nuclei oriented along long axis
  - Stretched epithelial bridging
  - Fenestrated appearance: Irregular, angulated or slit-like "holes"
- Crescentic residual lumen when florid
- Infrequent mitotic figures, may have intraductal necrosis

Grading Criteria
- Based on thickness of proliferation beyond 2 cell layer
- Mild: 3-4 cell layers thick ("non-proliferative" hyperplasia)
- Moderate: 5 or more cell layers thick, no duct distention
- Florid: Ducts distended and occluded by proliferation

Clinical Issues

Presentation
- No specific presentation; usually incidental finding
- Usually focal density or indeterminate microcalcifications

Natural History
- No consistent progression to malignancy

Treatment
- No specific treatment; chemoprevention not studied
- Annual or biennial mammography according to age
- Regular clinical and/or self-breast examination

Prognosis
- Mild IDH considered a normal variation
- Increased relative risk for malignancy
  - 1.5–2X above normal
  - Carcinoma in same quadrant, >10 years later
  - Unrelated to degree of hyperplasia
- Potential for risk stratification through molecular pathology

Selected References
1. Boecker W et al: Usual ductal hyperplasia of the breast is a committed stem (progenitor) cell lesion distinct from atypical ductal hyperplasia and ductal carcinoma in situ. J Pathol 198:458-67, 2002
2. Shaaban AM et al; Breast cancer risk in usual ductal hyperplasia is defined by estrogen receptor-alpha and Ki-67 expression. Am J Pathol 160:597-604, 2002
3. Bodian CA et al: Prognostic significance of benign proliferative breast disease. Cancer 71:3896-907, 1993

Imaging Artifacts

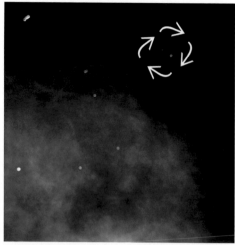

Imaging artifacts. Radiographic film artifact secondary to droplets in the cassette screen mimicking rounded microcalcifications on this magnification mammogram. Densities appear lucent centered but extend beyond the edge of the breast (arrows).

Key Facts
- Definition: Any physical, electronic, chemical or digital phenomenon that interferes with image interpretation
  - Mimics or obscures normal, or pathologic structures
- May be intrinsic to modality, procedure related, or extraneous to imaging process

Imaging Findings
<u>General Features</u>
- Best imaging clue: Appearance or finding that does not correspond to anatomy or range of pathology; typical appearance of common artifact
- Often obvious, but may mimic or obscure pathology
- Common to all modalities
  - Motion artifacts
  - Film artifacts
  - Image distortion
  - Image magnification
- Intrinsic to imaging modality
  - Due to physics of modality, positioning, technique, anatomy of patient
<u>Processor and Film-Related Artifacts</u>
- Any hard copy printed output, especially if processed conventionally
- Occur anywhere on film
- Roller marks: Linear fine or thick lines, usually lighter than image
- Stains and blotches: Film may be affected before or after exposure and processing (e.g., damp film)
- Scratches: Sharply-defined, irregular, linear defects in emulsion
- Static electricity: Jagged linear or star-like radiodense markings
- Poor processing: High fog levels, poor contrast, excessively dark or light

Imaging Artifacts

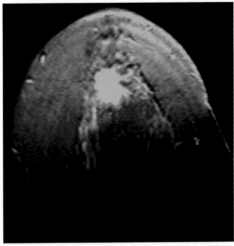

Imaging artifacts. Fat-suppressed post-gadolinium MRI in a woman with a large spiculated breast carcinoma, showing intense enhancement. Note variation of signal intensity across field from chest wall to nipple with differential fat suppression. Breast too large for coil design.

- o Improper temperature settings
- o Incorrect replenishment rate or processing time
- o Contaminated or exhausted developer
- o Improper film fixing and/or washing
- Raster artifacts: Horizontal linear misregistration (especially laser cameras)
- Faulty emulsion batch
- o Too dark or too light despite correct processor & exposure settings

Mammography Artifacts
- Procedure-related
  - o Poor positioning: Patient's hair, nose, chin, axillary fold
  - o Inadequate compression
  - o Motion blur
  - o Poor exposure
    - Incorrect automatic exposure chamber (AEC) positioning
    - Generator and power supply failures
- Mammography machine-related
  - o Incorrect collimation
  - o Grid inhomogeneity, stationary grid lines (Bucky failure)
  - o Compression system failure
- Film & screen-related
  - o Faulty screens: Variable density across image
  - o Quantum mottle: Mottled variation in radiographic density over moderately dense tissues
- Foreign material: Radiodense opacities which are usually recognizable, may mimic suspicious microcalcifications
  - o On screens: Fingerprints, dust, smoke particles, hair
  - o On cassettes: Contrast media, metallic particles
  - o On patient: Clothing, talc

Imaging Artifacts

o In patient: Pacemaker, tattoos, foreign bodies

Ultrasound Artifacts
- Refraction: Shadowing at edge of smoothly-marginated lesions
- Reverberation: Intracystic echoes paralleling cyst walls
- Specular reflection: Bright linear echo at center of superficial and deep surface of lesion; typical of benign smooth lesions
- Posterior enhancement: Increase in echogenicity and brightness deep to a structure; typical in cysts; some carcinomas (e.g., colloid)
- Shadowing: Reduction in echogenicity & brightness deep to a structure; often present in carcinomas
  - o Common but benign: Cooper's ligaments, scarring, fat necrosis, fibrosis, complex cysts

MR Artifacts
- Motion
  - o "Ghosting" replication artifacts in direction of phase encoding
    - ▪ Physiologic: Breathing, cardiac or vascular pulsation
    - ▪ Gross patient motion during sequence
  - o Gross patient motion between sequences: Produces subtraction artifacts which increase or obscure focal enhancement
- Fat suppression: Variation in image intensity after spectral fat suppression pulse; may suppress water instead
  - o Bulk susceptibility artifact
  - o Poor coil design
  - o Very large or very small breasts relative to coil
  - o Imperfect tuning of suppression pulse
  - o Field distortion due to metallic objects, (e.g., ports, implant valve)

Imaging Recommendations
- Recognition and awareness are crucial
- Change imaging parameters or plane
- Correct presumed problems and repeat imaging

Differential Diagnosis
Suspicious Microcalcifications on Mammography (Mimic DCIS)
- Artifacts usually too dense (e.g., dust) or regular (e.g., skin talc)

Suspicious Shadowing on Ultrasound (Mimic Carcinoma)
- May mimic neoplasm, focal lesion
- Confirm in multiple planes, correlate with known scars, etc.

Bright on Post-Contrast MRI (Mimic Carcinoma)
- Subtraction or suppression artifact

Pathology
- Careful attention required to differentiate imaging artifact from true lesion

Clincal Issues
- Any clinically suspicious findings not seen with imaging must be evaluated on clinical grounds alone

Selected References
1. Baker JA et al: Artifacts and pitfalls in sonographic imaging of the breast. AJR 176:1261-6, 2001
2. Coulthard A et al: Pitfalls of breast MRI. Br J Radiol 73:665-71, 2000
3. Hogge JP et al: Quality assurance in mammography: Artifact analysis. Radiographics 19:503-22, 1999

Intramammary Lymph Node

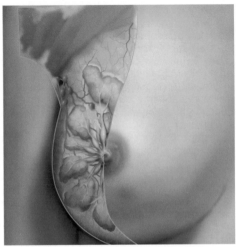

Intramammary lymph node. Cut-away drawing shows intramammary lymph node, axillary lymph nodes and lymphatic channels (in green). The most common location for intramammary lymph nodes is in the upper outer quadrant or the lateral breast.

Key Facts
- Synonym: Intraparenchymal lymph node
- Definition: Oval, smoothly-marginated, fat-containing mass
- Classic Imaging Appearance
  o Reniform or lobulated mass with a fatty hilum or notch
- Other Key Facts
  o Common
  o Lateral breast
  o Mammographic image usually diagnostic

Imaging Findings
Mammography Findings
- Reniform fat-containing mass
  o Radiolucent fat seen in periphery on tangential view
  o Fat seen centrally when en face
- < 1 cm
  o Size less important than classic appearance
- Lateral breast
  o Upper outer quadrant
  o May be anywhere in breast
  o May be multiple

MR Findings
- T1 C-: Small, smooth, well-circumscribed, fat-containing masses
- Post T1 C+: Mass enhances
  o Enhancement may be quite intense
  o Time/intensity curves may be suspicious for carcinoma
  o Lymphoid hyperplasia reported as rapid contrast uptake
  o Correlation with mammography/sonography helpful

Ultrasound Findings
- Hypoechoic oval mass, well circumscribed

Intramammary Lymph Node

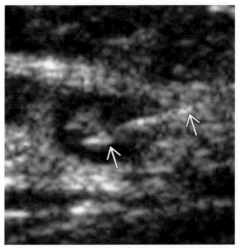

Intramammary lymph node. The smooth oval mass demonstrates a hypoechoic cortex and an echogenic fatty hilum. A biopsy needle (arrows) is seen within the cortex.

- o Lymphoidal tissue cortex
- Focal internal echogenicity
  - o Fat

Differential Diagnosis
Circumscribed Non-Calcified Mass
- No visible fat
- Nonspecific – large differential
- Ultrasound may benefit

Other Fat-Containing Well-Circumscribed Masses
- Encapsulated fat-containing masses are benign
- Typically do not require further imaging or intervention

Pathology
General
- Lymph node completely surrounded by breast tissue
- Lateral breast common location
- Enlargement
  - o Neoplasms
    - ▪ Breast cancer
    - ▪ Lymphoma
    - ▪ Melanoma
  - o Regional inflammation
    - ▪ Dermatitis
  - o Infections
    - ▪ Tuberculosis
    - ▪ Fungal
  - o Foreign body reaction
    - ▪ Gold injections
  - o Sinus histiocytosis

Intramammary Lymph Node

- Sinusoidal distention with histiocytes
- Immune reaction manifestation
- Marked sinusitis may confer improved prognosis in cancer patients

<u>Gross Pathologic, Surgical Features</u>
- Discrete, smooth, bean-shaped mass

<u>Microscopic Features</u>
- Fine needle aspiration
  - Lymphocytes
- Core biopsy
  - Capsule
  - Subcapsular sinuses

Clinical Issues

<u>Presentation</u>
- Nonpalpable, typically

<u>Treatment</u>
- No treatment unless suspicious imaging or clinical findings

<u>Prognosis</u>
- Excellent

Selected References
1. Rosen PP: Rosen's breast pathology. Lippincott Williams & Wikins, Philadelphia PA; chapter 45, 925-7, 2001
2. Kopans D: Breast imaging 2nd edition. Lippincott-Raven, Philadelphia PA; chapter 13, 273, 1998
3. Bassett LW et al: Diagnosis of diseases of the breast. Philadelphia: WB Saunders Co; chapter 25, 366-72, 1997

Juvenile Papillomatosis (JP)

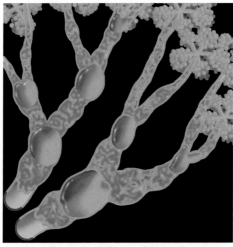

Drawing of juvenile papillomatosis. Multiple nodular papillomas arise in the TDLUs and are connected by ductal tissue, which contains papillary hyperplasia. Numerous small cysts are universally present.

Key Facts
- Synonym: Multiple papillomas, "Swiss-cheese" disease
- Definition: Multifocal proliferation of papillary tissue with fibrovascular stalks within multiple terminal ductal lobular units (TDLUs)
- Classic imaging appearance
  - Hypoechoic inhomogeneous mass on US with multiple small cysts
- Other key facts
  - Almost always in young women
  - Typically present as firm, multinodular, mobile mass

Imaging Findings
General Features
- Best imaging clue: Inhomogeneously hypoechoic, multinodular mass with cysts on US
- Shape – lobulated, multinodular, poorly defined
- Size range – 1 to 8 cm
Mammography Findings
- Nonspecific, focal, multinodular density
- With or without distortion
Ultrasound Findings
- Heterogeneous, hypoechoic, multinodular area with poorly-defined margins
- Multiple small cysts common, often around margins
MR Findings
- T1 C- – nodular hypointense lesion
- T2WI – multiple small hyperintense cysts
- T1 C+ – multilobulated, strongly-enhancing nodules
Imaging Recommendations
- Mammography not usually initially performed (young age)
- Ultrasound suggestive in appropriate clinical context

Juvenile Papillomatosis (JP)

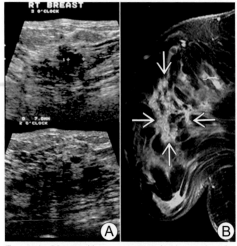

Juvenile papillomatosis. 26-year-old woman presented with a poorly-defined thickening in right breast. (A) Ultrasound shows a poorly-defined, multinodular, hypoechoic area with multiple small cysts. (B) Post T1 C+ MRI shows multifocal nodular intense enhancement connected by enhancing ducts (arrows).

- Imaging surveillance following treatment

Differential Diagnosis

Fibroadenoma
- Also mobile firm nodular mass in young woman
- Benign, stroma & epithelium

Papilloma
- Focal solitary papillary tumors with fibrovascular core
- Central or peripheral focal nodule or intracystic mass

Papillary Duct Hyperplasia (Aka Papillomatosis)
- Microscopic papillary hyperplasia in multiple ducts
- Children and young women, may present as mass
- Often solid, cysts not a feature

Pathology

General
- General Path Comments
  - First described 1980
  - 3D studies
    - Multifocal TDLU origin
    - Growth along interconnecting ducts
- Pathogenesis unknown
- Epidemiology
  - Young women < 30 years old
  - Uncommon before puberty and after 40
  - Very rare in males
  - Only small incidence of subsequent carcinoma if no family history
    - Increased risk of carcinoma in women with positive family history in maternal female relatives

Juvenile Papillomatosis (JP)

Gross Pathologic, Surgical Features
- Lobulated mass with multiple small cysts ("Swiss cheese")
- Intervening yellow or white flecks, mimic comedonecrosis

Microscopic Features
- Mixed spectrum of benign proliferative changes
- Cysts and ductal hyperplasia are invariable
- May show sclerosing adenosis, lobular or fibroadenomatoid hyperplasia
- May have cellular atypia
- Rarely associated carcinoma

Clinical Issues

Presentation
- Young woman with multinodular mobile, palpable breast mass
- Nipple discharge rarely present
- May have prior history of single or multiple benign breast biopsies

Natural History
- Not considered premalignant for most women
- May progress to carcinoma in up to 10% over 5-15 years, if maternal history of breast cancer
  o Genetic linkage not yet studied
- Can develop metachronous or contralateral disease

Treatment
- Complete surgical excision
- No further treatment if no malignancy found
- Treatment for malignancy if carcinoma found

Prognosis
- Recur in about 10%
  o Especially if bilateral or multifocal
- Patient should receive annual clinical examination and US
- Maternal female relatives should be regularly screened

Selected References
1. Mussurakis S et al: Case report: MR imaging of juvenile papillomatosis of the breast. Br J Radiol 69:867-70, 1996
2. Rosen PP et al: Juvenile papillomatosis of the breast. A follow-up study of 41 patients having biopsies before 1979. Am J Clin Pathol 93:599-603, 1990
3. Kersschot EA et al: Juvenile papillomatosis of the breast: Sonographic appearance. Radiology 169: 631-3, 1988

Lactating Adenoma

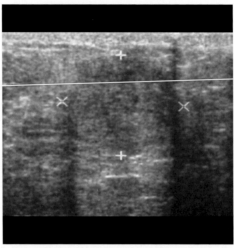

Lactating adenoma. 23-year-old woman noted enlarging right lower inner quadrant breast mass during pregnancy. Ultrasound examination performed four days postpartum revealed a well-defined, hypoechoic mass with posterior acoustic enhancement.

Key Facts
- Synonyms: Nodular lactational hyperplasia, lactating nodule
- Definition: Well-differentiated benign tumor of breast
  - Pregnant and lactating women
- Classic imaging appearance
  - Often indistinguishable from fibroadenoma
  - Can mimic malignancy
- Other key facts
  - Must be distinguished from carcinoma
    - 3% of breast cancers diagnosed in pregnancy
  - Usually involutes spontaneously after pregnancy or lactation
  - Most often occurs in anterior portion of breast
  - May be multiple

Imaging Findings
<u>General Features</u>
- Mammography not routinely recommended during pregnancy
  - Also, may be compromised during lactation
  - However, any highly suspicious finding must be evaluated
- Ultrasound helpful
  - Not diagnostic

<u>Mammography Findings</u>
- Well-circumscribed, round or oval mass
- Low or equal density with breast parenchyma
- 2-3 cm
  - May grow larger
- Atypical appearances
  - Irregular
  - Ill-defined
  - Spiculated

Lactating Adenoma

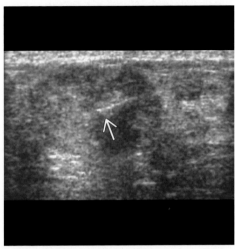

Lactating adenoma. Palpable mass in the right breast in a 40-year-old pregnant woman. Ultrasound examination revealed a well-circumscribed, hypoechoic mass with no accoustic enhancement. Ultrasound-guided core biopsy was performed. Note tip of 14-gauge tru-cut needle in center of mass (arrow).

Ultrasound Findings
- Oval, well-circumscribed, homogenous mass
- Low-level internal echoes
- Posterior acoustic enhancement
- Smooth lobulations
- Parallel to skin
- Echogenic pseudocapsule
- Less common
  o Angulated or ill-defined margins
  o Posterior acoustic shadowing

Imaging Recommendations
- Ultrasound imaging study of choice
- Mammography usually not indicated
  o Unless malignancy strongly suspected

Differential Diagnosis
Fibroadenoma
- Common in adolescents and women under 30
- Clinically smooth, firm or rubbery, and freely movable
- Hypoechoic, solid, well-circumscribed mass on ultrasound
- May have variable imaging characteristics

Galactocele
- Benign breast mass that contains retained milk
- Presentation may be delayed six to ten months after cessation of nursing
- Aspiration diagnostic and curative

Cyst
- Anechoic on ultrasound with posterior acoustic enhancement
- If equivocal, aspiration diagnostic

Lactating Adenoma

Well-Circumscribed Carcinoma
- Mimics benign lesions

Pathology
General
- Etiology-Pathogenesis
  - Origin controversial
    - De novo origin
    - Variant of preexisting tubular adenoma, fibroadenoma, or areas of lobular hyperplasia: Physiologic changes in pregnancy

Gross Pathologic, Surgical Features
- Circumscribed, grayish-white to yellow, firm and rubbery mass
- Becomes creamy yellow during lactation
- No true capsule
  - Sharply demarcated from surrounding breast tissue

Microscopic Features
- Florid lactational changes
- Tubuloalveolar appearance to glands

Cytological Features
- Loosely grouped clusters of epithelial cells with prominent nucleoli
- Foamy to vacuolated cytoplasm
- Atypia not seen

Clinical Issues
Presentation
- Palpable enlarging mass during pregnancy or lactation
- Mobile
  - May become fixed to overlying skin
- Diagnostic challenge

Natural History
- Majority of lesions regress spontaneously
- Infarction not uncommon
- Imaging findings not diagnostic
  - Fine needle aspiration biopsy or core biopsy recommended
  - Pathologist should be informed that patient is pregnant or lactating
    - Changes may be confused with carcinoma

Treatment
- No treatment usually necessary
- Surgical excision if mass does not resolve on its own

Prognosis
- Excellent
  - No malignant potential

Selected References
1. Behrndt VS: Infarcted lactating adenoma presenting as a rapidly enlarging breast mass. AJR 173:933-5, 1999
2. Scott-Conner CE: Breast cancer in pregnancy. Rosen Breast Cancer 30:595-601, 1999
3. Sumkin JH: Lactating adenoma: US features and literature review. Radiology 206:271-4, 1998

Lipoma

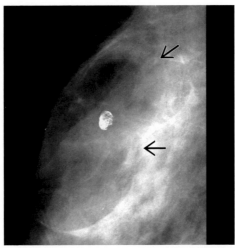

74-year-old woman with palpable upper outer quadrant left breast mass. Mammogram demonstrates an encapsulated, totally lucent mass (arrows) containing one coarse calcification with a lucent center consistent with fat necrosis. This lesion is consistent with a lipoma with a focus of calcified fat necrosis.

Key Facts
- Definition: Well-circumscribed, encapsulated, adipose tumor
- Classic Imaging Appearance
- Radiolucent circumscribed smooth mass surrounded with a thin dense capsule
- Other key facts
  - Common
  - Benign
    - No need for further imaging evaluation

Imaging Findings
Mammography Findings
- Lesions contain only fat
- Encapsulated lucent lesion
- Presence of fat on both sides of the capsule allows margin visibility
- Subject to necrosis
  - May exhibit typical spherical fat-containing calcifications
  - Margin may be spiculated due to fat necrosis
- May demonstrate surrounding architectural distortion
  - Secondary to tissue displacement
- No additional imaging is needed
MR Findings
- T1 C-: Bright, as these lesions contain fat
- Gadolinium enhanced: No enhancement
Ultrasound Findings
- Not necessary for characterization
- Hypoechoic
  - Similar to subcutaneous fat in breast
- Capsule may cause echo reflection
- Coarse calcifications may cause shadowing

Lipoma

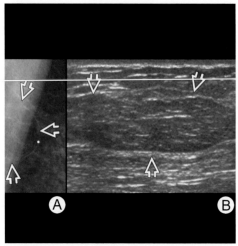

Lipoma. (A) Palpable mass in upper left breast (arrows). Totally composed of fat with a very thin capsule. (B) US directly over the palpable mass demonstrating an oval, smooth, well-circumscribed, hypoechoic mass. Note the essentially isoechoic nature of the mass as compared with the subcutaneous fat.

Differential Diagnosis

Benign Encapsulated Fat-Containing Lesions
- Hamartomas
  - o Typically have component of fibroglandular tissue
- Galactoceles
  - o Typically radiolucent, smoothly-margined masses
  - o Contain fat and inspissated secretions
  - o May demonstrate fat-fluid level on lateral mammogram
- Hibernoma
  - o Located in axillary tail or axilla
  - o Contain brown fat
- Fibrolipoma
  - o Mature adipose tissue and collagenous stroma

Oil Cysts
- Small, round, internally lucent masses with thin, calcified rims

Pathology

General
- Benign
- Usually single, well-circumscribed tumor with mature adipose tissue
- Usually unilateral
  - o Bilateral in 3%
- Multiple lipomas may occur
- Often in subcutaneous fat
- Fat necrosis may occur
  - o As with any fat-containing lesion

Gross Pathologic, Surgical Features
- Collections of fat

- May be firm with irregular margins
  o Secondary to fat necrosis

Microscopic Features
- Mature adipose cells

Clinical Issues

Presentation
- Mobile, generally soft
- May be somewhat firm
  o Secondary to fat necrosis

Treatment
- No treatment necessary

Selected References
1.   Rosen PP: Rosen's breast pathology. Lippincott Williams & Wikins, Philadelphia PA. Chapter 40, 786, 2001
2.   Kopans D: Breast imaging 2nd edition. Lippincott-Raven, Philadelphia PA. Chapter 19, 551-8, 1998
3.   Cardenosa G: Breast imaging companion. Lippincott-Raven, Philadelphia PA, 276, 1997

Mastitis

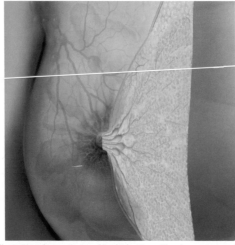

Mastitis. Illustration demonstrates skin thickening with edema represented by green fluid deep to the skin. Also suggested in the drawing is the hypertrophy of lymphatic system draining the infected breast.

Key Facts
- Synonyms: Breast infection, lactational mastitis
- Definition: Focal or diffuse breast infection usually related to lactation
- Classic mammographic appearance: Findings of edema
- Other key facts
  - Most common in lactating women
  - Staphylococcus aureus and streptococcal bacteria most common agents

Imaging Findings
Mammography Findings
- Not routinely performed
  - Clinical diagnosis
  - Young patient age
- Findings consistent with edema
  - Skin thickening
  - Trabecular coarsening
  - Overall increase in breast density
- Possible focal mass with abscess formation
Ultrasound Findings
- Diffuse or focal skin thickening
- Hypoechoic fluid in subcutaneous fat
- Hypoechoic mass = abscess
  - May have fluid-debris level
  - Air appears as echogenic specular reflectors with "dirty" shadowing
Imaging Recommendations
- Ultrasound for palpable and mammographic mass evaluation
- Typically a clinical management issue

Mastitis

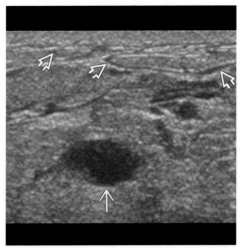

Mastitis. US from a lactating woman with erythematous, warm, painful breast shows mild skin thickening, hypoechoic fluid in subcutaneous fat (open arrows), and a portion of a dilated duct (arrow). The infectious process resolved with antibiotics.

Differential Diagnosis

Inflammatory Carcinoma
- Clinical and imaging findings may be indistinguishable
- Both entities may respond to antibiotic treatment
- Often requires punch skin biopsy for diagnosis

Non-Lactational Mastitis or Abscess Formation
- Fungal, parasitic, mycobacterial, viral, cat scratch disease
- Systemic or local treatment based on cultured agent
- Excision may be required

Subareolar Abscesses
- Nonlactating premenopausal women
- Duct obstruction
- Duct excision may be required

Granulomatous Mastitis
- Local inflammatory reaction
- Inspissated secretion or immune response

Lymphocytic Mastitis
- Accumulation of lymphocytes
- Local inflammatory reaction
- Inspissated secretion or immune response

Plasma Cell Mastitis
- Focal accumulation of plasma cells
- Local inflammatory reaction
- Inspissated secretion or immune response
- Rod-like "secretory" calcifications may develop

Mastitis

Pathology
<u>General</u>
- Bacterial entry via nipple
  - Contribution of stasis and duct obstruction
- Etiology-Pathogenesis
  - Staphylococcus more localized and invasive
  - Streptococcus more diffuse
    - Cellulitis
    - Abscesses in advanced cases
  - Abscesses may require drainage

<u>Gross Pathologic, Surgical Features</u>
- Diffuse breast inflammation
- Skin thickening
- Focal mass = abscess

<u>Microscopic Features</u>
- Leukocyte count > 10^6, bacterial count > 10^3
- Excised specimens mixed acute with chronic inflammation
- May have fat necrosis

Clinical Issues
<u>Presentation</u>
- Diffuse or focal breast changes
  - Edema
  - Erythema
  - Warmth
  - Pain
- Fever
- Possible focal mass
  - Abscess

<u>Treatment</u>
- Agent-specific antibiotics
- Drainage
- Possible surgical excision
  - Abscess

<u>Prognosis</u>
- Excellent

Selected References
1. Rosen PP: Rosen's breast pathology. Lippincott Williams & Wikins, Philadelphia PA; chapter 4, pg 65-75, 2001
2. Kopans D: Breast imaging 2nd edition. Lippincott-Raven, Philadelphia PA; chapter 19, 523-4, 1998
3. Bassett LW et al: Diagnosis of diseases of the breast. Philadelphia: WB Saunders Co; chapter 25, pp 382-5, 1997

Milk-Of-Calcium

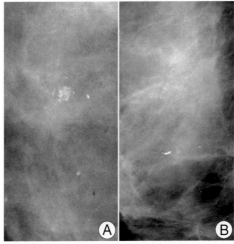

Milk-of-Calcium. (A) CC view of a cluster of somewhat hazy round calcifications. (B) True lateral mammograph showing that these calcifications are in a linear, almost meniscus-shaped, orientation consistent with layering in microcysts.

Key Facts
- Synonyms: Benign intracystic calcifications, sedimented calcifications
- Definition: Fine powdery calcifications precipitated into dilated lobules and microcysts
- Classic imaging appearance
  - "Pearls": Rounded, fuzzy, amorphous, calcific densities on CC
  - "Teacups": Sharply-defined crescentic or linear calcific shapes on horizontal beam views (LM, ML, prone, pendant)
- Other key facts
  - Always benign
  - Gravitationally dependent shapes
  - Freely mobile, powdery microcalcifications
  - May occur in large cysts

Imaging Findings
General Features
- Best imaging clue
  - Differing shapes of calcifications between CC and MLO views
- Shape
  - Rounded, "smudge-like" on CC view
  - Linear, semilunar or crescentic (concave upwards) on horizontal beam views
- Size range: 1–3 mm
- Location-center
  - Grouped, clustered or scattered through a segment
  - Usually in central to posterior glandular cone
  - Rare behind nipple, in accessory tissue or glandular islands
- Anatomy: Within dilated acini (microcysts)

Milk-Of-Calcium

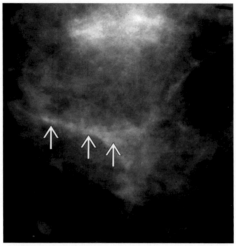

Milk-of-Calcium. This 45-year-old woman had hazy calcifications on her CC view that did not layer on diagnostic lateral mammogram. At the time of their stereotactic core biopsy, this prone scout view showed the calcifications in a linear (layering) orientation consistent with milk-of-calcium. The biopsy was canceled.

Mammography Findings
- Screening views: Differing shapes and density of calcifications between MLO and CC projections
- Grouped, or scattered, usually bilateral calcifications
- Special views
  o Horizontal beam views crucial to show mobile layering calcifications
  o LM and ML views usually diagnostic
  o Pendant and prone views sometimes required
- CC shows 1-2 mm, fuzzy, amorphous, rounded, calcific densities
- Horizontal beam views show
  o Denser well-defined calcifications
  o 2-3 mm crescentic (concave upwards) or linear densities
- Unusual appearances
  o Layering within macrocysts
  o Unilateral clustered distribution
  o "Sand-like" appearance on CC

Ultrasound Findings
- No specific findings

MR Findings
- No specific findings

Imaging Recommendations
- Suspect when calcifications differ in shape from view to view
  o Should have shapes corresponding to appropriate projections
- Perform appropriate horizontal beam films
- Perform prone views if necessary to confirm calcium layering

Differential Diagnosis
Ductal Carcinoma In Situ
- Heterogeneous or pleomorphic calcifications

- Grouped or clustered
- Not gravitationally dependent

Other Benign Calcifications
- Rounded, quite homogeneous shapes
- Shapes similar from view to view
- May be grouped or scattered
- Not gravitationally dependent

Pathology

General
- General Path Comments
  o Rarely associated with malignancy
  o Contained within dilated microcysts
- Etiology-Pathogenesis
  o Unknown
- Epidemiology
  o Usually postmenopausal
  o 4% of symptomatic women

Gross Pathologic, Surgical Features
- No specific features

Microscopic Features
- Dilated microcysts with tiny punctate calcifications
- Calcifications may not be visible (lost in specimen preparation)
- Rarely associated findings
  o Lipid cysts
  o Galactoceles
  o Adjacent malignancy (presumably incidental)

Clinical Issues

Presentation
- Usually incidental finding
- Screening mammography
- May present with lump or nipple discharge
  o Symptoms require further evaluation

Treatment
- No specific treatment
- Reassurance and routine screening
- May require needle biopsy for confirmation

Prognosis
- Always benign in isolation
- Rarely has adjacent malignancy; suspect if
  o Other more suspicious calcifications
  o Soft-tissue masses

Selected References
1. Moy L et al: The pendent view: An additional projection to confirm the diagnosis of milk of calcium. AJR 177:173-5, 2001
2. Ross BA et al: Milk of calcium in the breast: Appearance on prone stereotactic imaging. Breast J 7:53-5, 2001
3. Linden SS et al: Sedimented calcium in benign breast cysts: The full spectrum of mammographic presentations. AJR 152:967-71, 1989

Mondor's Disease

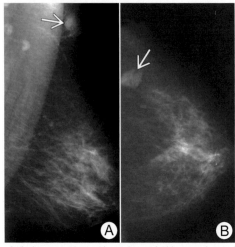

(A & B) Mondor's disease patient with painless palpable mass (arrows) unchanged over a number of years. The bluish-green mass was visible through the skin.

Key Facts
- Definition: Superficial thrombophlebitis
- Benign self-limited process
- A clinical diagnosis
- If calcified, vein is visible near skin on mammogram
- Usually associated with trauma, surgery, excessive exercise, injections
- May be associated with carcinoma (usually breast)
- Rarely associated with deep venous thrombosis

Imaging Findings
Mammography Findings
- Serpiginous tubular structure
  - May be beaded in appearance
- When calcified
  - Tram-track appearance
  - Typical for vascular calcification
Ultrasound Findings
- Dilated superficial tubular structure
- No Doppler flow
- Entire vessel course may be visible
  - Internal echoes
    - Thrombus
  - Anechoic
    - Multiple areas of narrowing
    - Beaded appearance

Differential Diagnosis
Tubular Structure (Single Dilated Duct)
- Typically intramammary and retroareolar locations
Collagen-Vascular Disease
- Dermatomyositis

Mondor's Disease

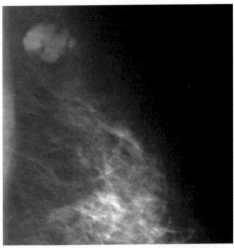

Mondor's disease. The multi-lobulated, smoothly-marginated mass (same mass as previous page) is better seen on this exaggerated CC view. While not truly serpiginous, the multi lobulated nature is consistent with a tortuous dilated vessel.

- o Vascular calcification associated with soft tissue calcification
- o Differentiate skin from vascular calcifications
- o Other collagen-vascular diseases
  - Prominent systemic manifestations differentiate

Pathology
General
- Self-limited condition of superficial veins
  - o Upper outer or inframammary breast and chest wall
- Etiology
  - o Trauma
  - o Surgery
  - o Excessive exercise
  - o Injections
  - o Jellyfish bites
  - o Pregnancy complication
  - o Carcinoma (breast and lung)

Gross Pathologic, Surgical Features
- Thrombosed, thickened vein

Microscopic Features
- Venous thrombosis
- Varying stages of organization and recanalization
- Mild inflammation of surrounding tissue

Clinical Issues
Presentation
- Young patient
  - o 20-40 years of age
- Painful mass
- Painless superficial cord

Mondor's Disease

- Painless mass
- Thoracoepigastric, lateral thoracic, or superior epigastric veins
- Both breasts equally affected
- 25% in men

Natural History
- Self-limited

Treatment
- Symptomatic treatment
- Biopsy avoided with careful assessment of clinical and imaging findings

Prognosis
- Excellent
  - Most cases resolve
  - Chronic thrombosis may lead to dense vascular calcifications

Selected References
1. Rosen PP: Rosen's breast pathology. Lippincott Williams & Wikins, Philadelphia PA; chapter 3, 48, 2001
2. Shetty MK et al: Mondor's disease of the breast; sonographic and mammographic findings. AJR 177:893-6, 2001
3. Bassett LW et al: Philadelphia: WB Saunders Co; Chapter 25, 364-6, 1997

Myoepithelial Neoplasms

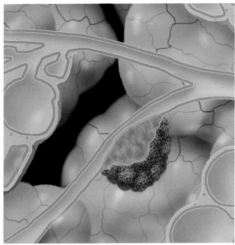

Adenomyoepithelioma, a benign focal myoepithelial neoplasm. A small, well-circumscribed mass is shown arising from abnormally proliferative and hyperplastic myoepithelial cells. Note the eccentric origin from the wall of a breast duct.

Key Facts
- Definition: Benign or malignant neoplasms arising from myoepithelial cells
- Classic imaging appearance
  - Focal nodular mass with clustered dense microcalcifications
- 5 entities: Dominant or pure myoepithelial origin (descending frequency)
  - Adenomyoepithelioma, benign or malignant
  - Myoepitheliosis (no imaging correlate)
  - Malignant myoepithelioma (myoepithelial carcinoma - extremely rare)
  - Pleomorphic adenoma (extremely rare)
  - Adenoid cystic carcinoma (extremely rare)

Imaging Findings
General Features
- Best imaging clue: Focal nodular mass with some dense calcifications
- Mostly nonspecific; myoepitheliosis not distinguishable from glandular parenchyma
- Shape: Nodular or lobulated, fairly well-defined margins
- Size range: 1–7 cm (adenomyoepithelioma), 1–20 cm (malignant myoepithelioma)
- Location: Anywhere in breast; adenomyoepithelioma central
Mammography Findings
- Nonspecific, well-defined mass or asymmetric density
- Microcalcifications, esp. adenomyoepithelioma
Ultrasound Findings
- Focal well-defined mass, usually hypoechoic
MR Findings
- No published descriptions
Imaging Recommendations
- Mammography and ultrasound best
- Image-guided core biopsy diagnostic

Myoepithelial Neoplasms

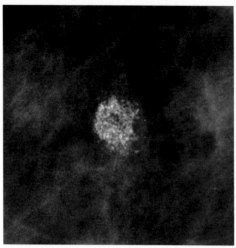

Myoepithelial neoplasms. Magnification view of a calcified right breast mass. Tightly clustered, very dense, atypical microcalcifications with slightly variable size, rounded shapes, and irregular margins are seen. Benign adenomyoepithelioma without atypia was found at core biopsy.

Differential Diagnosis
Fibroadenoma
- Nodular mass with dense microcalcifications
  - Calcifications coarser, peripheral distribution
- Much more common, usually younger women

Phyllodes Tumor
- When presenting with large rapidly growing mass
- Calcifications very uncommon in phyllodes tumor

Papilloma, Peripheral
- Nodular mass with dense microcalcifications
- Similar age range, size and location
- Cannot reliably distinguish without biopsy

Ductal Carcinoma
- Tubular, papillary and other uncommon variants if small
- NOS ductal carcinoma when large
- May coexist with adenomyoepithelioma
- Cannot reliably distinguish without biopsy

Pathology
General
- General Path Comments
  - Myoepithelial cells between ductal epithelium and basement membrane
  - Myoepitheliosis usually incidental finding at histology
  - Benign adenomyoepithelioma may show marked atypia on cytology
  - Firm rubbery masses with areas of cystic, hyaline or hemorrhagic degeneration
- Etiology-Pathogenesis
  - Unknown

Myoepithelial Neoplasms

- Epidemiology
  - Quite uncommon (adenomyoepithelioma) to extremely rare
  - Women, age 25–85, median 50-70

Gross Pathologic, Surgical Features

- Adenomyoepithelioma
  - Circumscribed round or multilobulated
- Myoepitheliosis
  - Firm irregular area, no mass
- Malignant myoepithelioma
  - Smooth or stellate, satellite nodules

Microscopic Features

- Abnormally proliferative and hyperplastic myoepithelial cells
- Myoepitheliosis – intraductal or periductal
  - Microscopic multifocal myoepithelial proliferation
- Adenomyoepithelioma – spindle, tubular or lobulated variants
  - Usually encapsulated, often marginal irregularity
  - Differentiate from tubular, ductal adenomas or sclerosing papilloma
- Malignant myoepithelioma – pure spindle cell malignancy

Staging or Grading Criteria

- Atypia not uncommon, does not indicate malignancy
- Carcinoma or sarcoma arising in adenomyoepithelioma is unequivocally malignant

Clinical Issues

Presentation

- Myoepitheliosis: No focal clinical findings
- Others
  - Usually palpable, focal, nodular mass, may be tender
  - May be detected on screening mammography (mass with calcifications)

Natural History

- Adenomyoepithelioma may be unchanged for years
  - Malignant transformation may occur
  - Marked increase in size if malignant
- Malignant adenomyoepithelioma
  - Metastasizes hematogenously
  - May spread to axillary nodes
- Other lesions: Prognosis unknown

Treatment

- Complete surgical excision curative; may recur locally
- Axillary node dissection usually unnecessary

Prognosis

- Malignant adenomyoepithelioma
  - No metastases reported if < 2 cm at surgery
  - Metastases to lung, thyroid, bone, poor prognosis
- Benign lesions: Good if completely excised

Selected References
1. Howlett DC et al: Adenomyoepithelioma of the breast: Spectrum of disease with associated imaging and pathology. AJR 180:799-803, 2003
2. Doyle AJ et al: Myoepithelial lesions of the breast: Imaging characteristics and diagnosis with large-core needle biopsy in two cases. Radiology 193:787-8, 1994
3. Tavassoli FA: Myoepithelial lesions of the breast. Myoepitheliosis, adenomyoepithelioma, and myoepithelial carcinoma. Am J Surg Pathol 15:554-68, 1991

Myoid Hamartoma

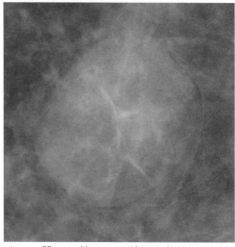

Myoid hamartoma.   55-year-old woman with an enlarging mammographic well-circumscribed mass surrounded by a lucent halo.   US guided core biopsy revealed a myoid lesion.   The patient elected to have the mass excised with histologic diagnosis of myoid hamartoma.

Key Facts
- Synonyms: Leiomyomatous hamartoma, muscular hamartoma
- Definition: Benign proliferative lesion
- Classic imaging appearance
  - Well-circumscribed mammographic mass
  - Lucent halo may be prominent
- Other key facts
  - Hyperechoic, well-circumscribed sonographic mass
  - Core biopsy findings may be difficult to differentiate from infiltrating lobular carcinoma

Imaging Findings
Mammography Findings
- Well-circumscribed round or oval mass
- May have lucent halo
- Heterogeneous density
Ultrasound Findings
- Well-circumscribed mass
- Internal echogenicity
  - May be complex

Differential Diagnosis
Infiltrating Lobular Carcinoma
- Epithelioid differentiation of myoepithelial cells may mimic infiltrating lobular carcinoma (ILC)
- A potential pitfall on core biopsy
  - Secondary to limited sampling
Circumscribed Carcinomas
- Medullary
- Mucinous

Myoid Hamartoma

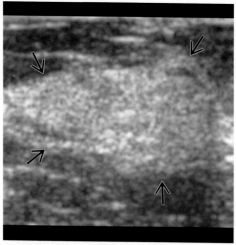

Myoid hamartoma. Sonogram from same woman demonstrates a well-circumscribed, oval, markedly hyperechoic mass (arrows).

- Infiltrating ductal carcinoma, not otherwise specified (NOS)
  - Unusual presentation as a circumscribed mass

Circumscribed Benign Lesions
- Cysts
- Fibroadenomas

Pathology
General
- Proliferative benign lesion
- Bands of smooth muscle, ducts, lobules and stroma
- Not a true hamartoma
  - Adenosis-type tumor with leiomyomatous myoid metaplasia

Gross Pathologic, Surgical Features
- Well-circumscribed fibrous mass
- Adipose tissue typically not evident
- May contain cysts with brown fluid

Microscopic Features
- Bundles of smooth muscle cells
  - Varying amounts of glandular and fibrous elements
- Foci of sclerosing adenosis common
- Immunohistochemistry supports myoepithelial cellular origin

Clinical Issues
Presentation
- Palpable
- May be image detected
- Size range 2-11 cm
- Upper outer quadrant predominance

Treatment
- May be adequately diagnosed with core biopsy
- No tendency for recurrence

Myoid Hamartoma

- No tendency for multifocality
- No tendency for bilaterality

Selected References
1. Rosen PP: Rosen's breast pathology. Lippincott Williams & Wikins, Philadelphia PA; chapter 40, 782-3, 2001
2. Garfein CF et al: Epithelioid cells in myoid hamartoma of the breast; a potential diagnostic pitfall for core biopsies. Arch Pathol Lab Med 121:354-5; 1997
3. Daroca PJ Jr et al: Myoid hamartomas of the breast. Hum Pathol 16:212-9, 1985

Oil Cyst

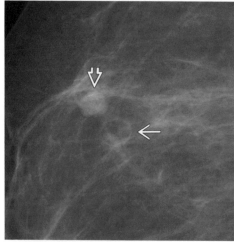

Oil cyst. 61-year-old woman with history of reduction mammoplasty. Well-circumscribed, noncalcified, fat-containing mass with a thin rim (arrow). The rim is visible because fat is present within and outside the mass. The oil cyst is adjacent to an intramammary lymph node (open arrow).

Key Facts
- Definition: Round to oval encapsulated lesion containing liquefied fat
- Manifestation of post-traumatic fat necrosis
- Commonly occurs secondary to breast trauma
  - Iatrogenic
    - Biopsy
    - Lumpectomy
    - Post-mastectomy TRAM flap reconstruction
    - Reduction mammoplasty (miminized with free nipple graft technique)
  - Injury
    - Blunt trauma
    - Penetrating trauma
    - Seatbelt injury
- Single or multiple
- All age groups
- Most common sites
  - Subareolar region
  - Superficial tissues near skin
- Not all cases thought to arise from fat necrosis
  - Steatocystoma multiplex
    - Round, well-circumscribed, intradermal masses
    - Intradermal oil cysts
    - Usually in adolescent or young men

Imaging Findings
Mammography Findings
- Well-circumscribed mass
  - May be calcified

Oil Cyst

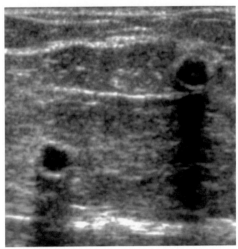

Oil cyst. 46-year-old asymptomatic woman with history of excisional biopsy of the left breast. Mammography demonstrated oil cysts at biopsy site. Ultrasound identified two of these lesions as well-defined, hypoechoic masses with posterior acoustic shadowing.

Ultrasound Findings
- Round to oval
- Usually anechoic
  o Variable posterior acoustic features
- May be hypoechoic or isoechoic
  o Variable posterior acoustic features
- Occasionally complex
  o Internal echogenic bands
  o Mural nodules

MR Findings
- High signal intensity on all pulse sequences
  o Except fat-saturated
- Moderate capsular enhancement with contrast agent

Imaging Recommendations
- Mammography

Differential Diagnosis

Steatocystoma Multiplex
- Rare cutaneous disorder
- Autosomal dominant
- Usually in adolescent or young men
- Multiple cutaneous intradermal cysts
  o Mainly trunk, upper extremities
- Usually asymptomatic
  o May become secondarily inflamed
- Soft to firm and smooth

Lipoma
- Circumscribed fat-containing lesion

Oil Cyst

- Soft and freely movable
- Asymptomatic
- Usually unilateral
- Mammography is diagnostic in most cases
  - Well-defined radiolucent mass
  - May have areas of fat necrosis
  - Thin radiopaque capsule
    - Usually does not calcify
- Ultrasound
  - Hypoechoic to isoechoic mass
  - Thin, echogenic capsule

Pathology
Gross Pathological, Surgical Features
- Thick, oily material obtained at aspiration or surgery

Clinical Issues
Presentation
- Often asymptomatic
  - Detected on screening mammography
- May present as tender palpable mass or masses
- Reduction mammoplasty
  - Often develops beneath scars
Treatment
- No treatment necessary
- Biopsy not necessary if meets imaging criteria for oil cyst
Prognosis
- Excellent
  - No malignant potential

Selected References
1. Bilgen, IG et al: Fat necrosis of the breast: Clinical, Mammographic and Sonographic Features. EurJourRad 39(2):92-99, 2001
2. Soo, MS: Fat necrosis in the breast: Sonographic Features. Radiology. 206:261-96, 1998
3. Hogge, JP et al: The mammographic spectrum of fat necrosis of the breast. Radiographics. 15:1347-56, 1995

Papilloma

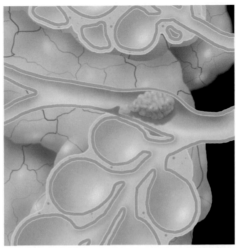

Papilloma. Diagram depicts a representation of a papillary intraductal mass supported by a stalk. Note that the duct in this case is dilated. The clinical setting in such a case as shown here might be spontaneous bloody nipple discharge.

Key Facts
- Synonyms: Large duct papilloma, intraductal papilloma, intracystic papilloma, central papilloma
- Definition: Benign ductal neoplasm with papillary growth pattern supported by a fibrovascular stalk
- Classic imaging appearance
  - Periareolar intraluminal soft-tissue mass
- Other key facts
  - Majority present with bloody nipple discharge
  - "Intracystic" = within hugely dilated duct
  - Not malignant or premalignant
  - Associated with slight increased risk of developing breast cancer
  - Distinguish from papillomatosis
    - Form of epithelial hyperplasia

Imaging Findings
General Features
- Other features
  - Shape = Oval or round
  - Size range = 0.5-3 cm
  - Location = Central 70-90%
- Anatomy
  - Central, periareolar
    - Usually solitary
    - Intraductal or intracystic
  - Peripheral
    - Any quadrant; solitary or multiple
    - Arise from terminal ductal lobular unit (TDLU)
Mammography Findings
- Usually not visible

Papilloma

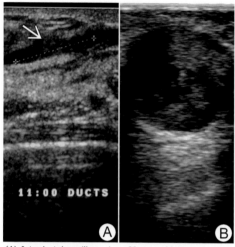

Papilloma. (A) Intraductal papilloma in a 32-year-old woman with bloody nipple discharge. Dilated lactiferous duct with intraluminal solid tissue (arrow). (B) Intracystic papilloma in a 56-year-old woman with a palpable periareolar mass. Well-defined complex cystic lesion containing a lobulated soft tissue mass.

- May present as a nonspecific mass
- Sclerosing papilloma may be spiculated
  - Mimics carcinoma
- May have microcalcifications
  - Large, irregular, dense, grouped
  - "Shell-like," lucent-centered
- Galactography
  - Focal intraductal filling defect
- Pneumocystography
  - Focal intracystic nodular mass

Ultrasound Findings
- Retroareolar angled, "rolled nipple" imaging technique
- Focal hypoechoic solid mass
  - Well-defined, usually lobulated mass
  - Cystic lesion with internal solid components
  - Dilated ducts around lesion common

MR Findings
- T1 C- & T2WI – nonspecific, isointense, soft-tissue mass
- T1 C+ – usually weak enhancement
- Not specific enough to reliably distinguish benign from malignant

Imaging Recommendations
- US-guided core or vacuum-assisted biopsy diagnostic
- Galactography
  - Confirms intraluminal tumor

Differential Diagnosis
Papillary Carcinoma
- Usually intracystic or nodular
- Lacks myoepithelial membrane

Papilloma

- Cannot be distinguished from papilloma on cytology
Papillomatosis
- Form of epithelial hyperplasia
- Typically in peripheral ducts
- Children, adolescents and young adults

Pathology
General
- General Comments
  o Frozen section may misdiagnose as carcinoma
  o May be found adjacent to papillary carcinoma
  o May have cellular atypia
  o May show marked sclerosis, metaplasia
- Epidemiology
  o Females > 50 years old
  o Rare in adolescents, young adults
Gross Pathologic, Surgical Features
- Dilated duct with mural soft-tissue mass
- Mass may obliterate lumen
Microscopic Features
- Dilated duct around mass
- Epithelial fronds with fibrovascular stroma
- Myoepithelial cell layer
  o Between epithelial cells and basement membrane
- Hemorrhagic infarction of fronds common

Clinical Issues
Presentation
- Bloody nipple discharge in majority
- Occasionally clinically palpable mass
Natural History
- May undergo spontaneous infarction
Treatment
- When diagnosed by core biopsy (follow-up controversial)
  o Surgical excision vs imaging follow-up
  o Excise when papilloma associated with malignancy, atypia
- When suggested with galactography
  o Localize lesion and surgically excise
- When found by ultrasound
  o Ultrasound-guided mammotome excision (controversial)
Prognosis
- Cured if completely excised
- < 10% recurrence rate

Selected References
1. Dennis MA et al: Incidental treatment of nipple discharge caused by benign intraductal papilloma through diagnostic mammotome biopsy. AJR 174:1263-8, 2000
2. Orel SG et al: MR imaging in patients with nipple discharge: Initial experience. Radiology 216:248-54, 2000
3. Yang WT et al: Sonographic features of benign papillary neoplasms of the breast: Review of 22 patients. J Ultrasound Med 16:161-8, 1997

PASH

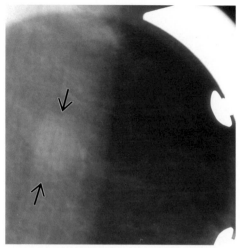

PASH. Spot compression image from a 48-year-old's screening mammogram demonstrates a new upper outer quadrant, round, fairly well-circumscribed mass without calcifications or associated findings (arrows). Excisional biopsy diagnosed PASH and fibrocystic changes. (Courtesy of Elizabeth Rafferty, MD).

Key Facts
- Synonym: Pseudoangiomatous stromal hyperplasia (PASH)
- Definition: Benign neoplastic myofibroblastic process
- Other key facts
  - Uncommon
  - Mean size 5-6 cm
  - Premenopausal women
  - Histologically distinctive myofibroblast-lined slit-like spaces
  - May be incidental diffuse pathologic entity or focal finding

Imaging Findings
Mammography Findings
- Round or oval mass
  - Noncalcified
  - 1-10 cm
  - Margins fairly well circumscribed
    - Indistinct
    - Obscured

Ultrasound Findings
- Round or oval mass
- Variable margin characteristics
- Variable internal echogenicity
  - Hypoechoic
  - Hyperechoic
  - Mixture
- Posterior echo pattern variable
  - Shadowing
  - Enhancement

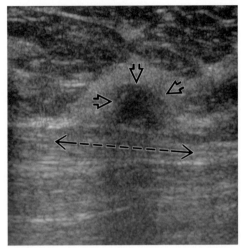

PASH. Ultrasound of the same case, demonstrates an irregular 1.8 cm hypoechoic mass not parallel to the skin with indistinct margins (open arrows) and echogenic rim. The mass is located immediately anterior to the pectoralis muscle (double headed arrow). (Courtesy of Elizabeth Rafferty, MD).

MR Findings
- T1 C-
  - Intermediate signal with interspersed lower signals
- T2WI
  - Mixed high and low signal
- T1 C+
  - Intense wall enhancement of cystic component

Differential Diagnosis
Low Grade Angiosarcoma
- A true vasoformative lesion
Fibroadenoma
- Usually smaller
  - 2-3 cm
- Cellular findings may be similar
- Stromal characteristics helpful
Phyllodes
- Cellular aspirates may limit correct diagnosis
Hamartoma
- Similar hyperplastic changes
- No myofibroblastic-lined stromal spaces
- Fat-containing
- Reports of PASH cases misdiagnosed as hamartomas

Pathology
General
- A benign mesenchymal lesion
- Diffuse or focal stromal changes
  - Characteristic anastomosing slit-like stromal spaces

PASH

- Fine needle aspiration may be inconclusive
  - Epithelial component appears more prominent
  - Surgical excision may be required for definitive diagnosis
- Nonspecific proliferative epithelial changes
- Etiology-Pathogenesis
  - Typically premenopausal women
  - Hormonal influence
  - Postmenopausal women
    - Hormone replacement
    - Nonpalpable forms may be mammographically visible

Gross Pathologic, Surgical Features
- Focal lesions
  - Smooth, well-demarcated surface
- May contain cysts
  - < 1 cm

Microscopic Features
- Striking stromal changes
  - Complex anastomosing pattern of spaces
  - Separation of stromal collagen fibers
  - Lining cells
    - Fibroblasts
    - Myofibroblasts
  - No endothelial cells
- Epithelial elements
  - Lobular and ductal structures
  - May show proliferative changes

Clinical Issues
Presentation
- Premenopausal
  - Palpable, unilateral, painless, firm or rubbery mass
- Postmenopausal
  - Mammographic mass in woman taking hormone replacement
- Microscopic findings seen in gynecomastia
- Reported in axillary tissue
- Immunosuppressed patients

Natural History
- May show rapid growth
  - Requires biopsy for differentiation from neoplasm

Treatment
- Wide local excision

Prognosis
- Excellent
  - Local recurrences reported

Selected References
1. Kirkpatrick UJ et al: Imaging appearance of pseudoangiomatous hyperplasia of mammary stroma. Clin Radiol 55:576-8, 2000
2. Piccoli CW et al: Developing asymmetric breast tissue. Radiology 211:111-7, 1999
3. Vicandi B et al: Nodular pseudoangiomatous stromal hyperplasia of the breast: Cytologic features. Acta Cytol 42:335-41, 1998

Phyllodes Tumor

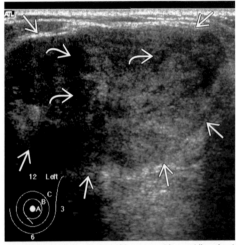

Phyllodes tumor. Ultrasound of a 40-year-old woman with a rapidly enlarging, palpable, 6 cm mass in the lower left breast. The tumor is smoothly marginated (arrows), solid and moderately hypoechoic with heterogeneous areas of lower echogenicity (curved arrows).

Key Facts
- Synonyms: Cystosarcoma phyllodes, periductal stromal tumor
- Definition: Circumscribed connective tissue and epithelial neoplasm from periductal stroma with leaf-like proliferation into cystic spaces
- Classic imaging appearance: Very large smoothly marginated breast mass without calcifications
- Other key facts
  - Benign (40-80%), borderline (10-20%) or malignant (5-30%)
  - May metastasize
  - High-grade phyllodes tumor 5-year survival rate 55-75%

Imaging Findings
General Features
- Best imaging clue: Large smoothly marginated mass
- Shape: Lobulated, round or oval
- Size range: 1-45 cm, mean size 4-5 cm, may occupy entire breast
- Cannot distinguish from giant fibroadenoma
- Cannot distinguish benign, borderline or malignant
Mammography Findings
- Dense, smoothly-marginated or lobulated round or oval mass
- Microcalcifications rare
Ultrasound Findings
- Ovoid or round, smoothly-marginated hypoechoic, mass
- Sound transmission decreased, isoechoic or increased
- Homogeneous, may have intramural cystic foci
MR Findings
- T1 C- & T2WI – nonspecific, large, lobulated mass
- T1 C+ – rapidly-enhancing, lobulated mass, no washout

Phyllodes Tumor

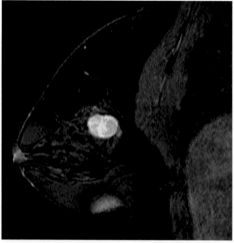

Phyllodes tumor. Sagittal fat-suppressed T1 C+ MRI of benign phyllodes tumor. Smoothly-marginated, intensely enhancing nodule with some internal heterogeneity. This appearance is indistinguishable from a fibroadenoma.

Differential Diagnosis
Giant Fibroadenoma (GFA)
- Occurs in younger women typically
- No significant malignant potential
- Less cellular stroma
- Lack of leaf-like proliferation, cysts

Pathology
General
- General Path Comments
  - Arises from periductal stroma
  - Minority have significant malignant potential
  - Even benign may recur locally
  - Needle biopsy useful preoperatively
    - Fine needle > 92% accuracy for diagnosis
    - Core needle or excision biopsy for grading
- Genetics
  - No hereditary factors
- Etiology-Pathogenesis
  - Unknown
- Epidemiology
  - Almost exclusively women
  - Age range 10-80, rare < 30 or > 60
  - Median age 45-49
Gross Pathologic, Surgical Features
- Solid, fleshy mass with bulging surface, cystic areas
- Well-circumscribed, nonencapsulated
- Gray to yellow foci of necrosis and hemorrhage
Microscopic Features
- Benign epithelial component

Phyllodes Tumor

- Cellular spindle cell fibroblastic stroma
- Leaf-like processes protruding into cystic spaces
- Highly atypical or multinucleated giant cells may occur
- Metaplasia (lipoid, chondroid, osteoid) may occur
- P53 immunohistochemical staining
  - o Focal in benign, more diffuse in borderline & malignant
  - o May be absent in many malignant phyllodes

Staging or Grading Criteria (AFIP)
- Low grade – pushing margin, mild atypia, < 3 mitoses/high power field (hpf); usually smaller
- High grade – infiltrative margin, moderate to severe atypia, $\geq$ 3 mitoses/hpf
- Metaplastic malignancy within phyllodes rare (sarcoma, carcinoma)

Clinical Issues
Presentation
- Woman in middle age with firm, mobile, palpable lump
  - o Older age group than fibroadenoma (median 45-49, rare under 30)
  - o Lump may show rapid growth over few weeks
  - o No pain, bleeding
  - o Skin may be stretched or ulcerated (pressure effect)

Treatment
- Complete surgical excision often curative
  - o Margin $\geq$ 1 cm to minimize recurrence
  - o Wide local excision required
  - o Mastectomy for very large tumors
  - o Axillary node dissection unnecessary
- Features predisposing local recurrence
  - o Incomplete excision and invasive tumor border
- Adjuvant therapy
  - o Radiotherapy reduces local recurrence
  - o No benefit from chemotherapy

Prognosis
- If wide local excision
  - o Local recurrence uncommon for benign (< 10% over 10 years)
  - o Higher rate for borderline (29%) and malignant (36%)
- 5-year survival for malignant phyllodes = 55-75%

Selected References
1. Yilmaz E et al: Differentiation of phyllodes tumors versus fibroadenomas. Acta Radiol 43:34-9, 2002
2. Veneti S et al: Benign phyllodes tumor vs. fibroadenoma: FNA cytological differentiation. Cytopathology 12:321-8, 2001
3. Barth RJ Jr: Histologic features predict local recurrence after breast conserving therapy of phyllodes tumors. Breast Cancer Res Treat 57:291-5, 1999

Round Punctate Calcifications

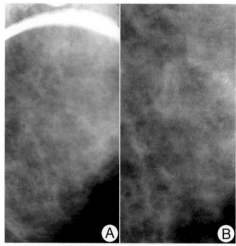

Spot compression view of punctate, tiny, rounded calcifications. (A) Calcifications are seen as faint tiny opacities. (B) Detail view of the same area shows them to be extremely small and sharply defined. Proven benign at needle biopsy.

Key Facts
- Synonyms
  - Lobular calcifications
  - Acinar calcifications
- Definition
  - Tiny, focal, sharply-defined calcifications, either grouped or scattered
- Classic imaging appearance
  - Focal group of tiny, round or oval, sharply-defined calcifications
- Other key facts
  - Usually screen detected
  - Asymptomatic
  - Occasionally associated with malignancy if mixed with pleomorphic heterogeneous calcifications

Imaging Findings
General Features
- Shape
  - Round or oval
- Size range
  - 0.1 – 0.5 mm
- Location
  - Anywhere in glandular tissue
  - Rarely isolated away from glandular cone
Mammography Findings
- Tiny, sharply-defined calcifications
- Rounded or oval contours
- May have slight shape heterogeneity
- Usually grouped, sometimes scattered
- May be in multiple groups
- May be intermixed with heterogeneous calcifications

Round Punctate Calcifications

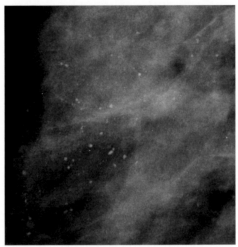

Very high magnification view of benign microcalcifications showing tiny, punctate, less dense microcalcifications intermixed with denser, benign, smooth, rounded microcalcifications. There are no suspicious features.

- o More likely to have associated malignancy
- Appearance may change on serial mammography
- o Increase or decrease number

Ultrasound Findings
- No abnormality
- Calcifications usually too small to detect

MR Findings
- No specific findings

Imaging Recommendations
- Magnification views required for adequate assessment
- Typical appearance can be dismissed
- Intermixed heterogeneous calcifications may indicate malignancy

Differential Diagnosis
Skin Talc
- Usually typical distribution in skin pores
- Minimize through appropriate patient instruction
- Occasionally confounding

Sclerosing Adenosis
- May have clustered or diffuse calcifications
- May have associated focal mass or density
- Ultrasound may show lobulated or shadowing mass

Pathology
General
- General Path Comments
  - o Not specific for particular pathologic finding
- Etiology-Pathogenesis

Round Punctate Calcifications

- o Usually in dilated acini and lobules
- Epidemiology
  - o Uncommon under 40
  - o Common on screening mammography

Gross Pathologic, Surgical Features
- No specific features

Microscopic Features
- Dilated lobular acini-containing calcifications
- Type I microcalcifications
  - o Calcium oxalate crystals
  - o Birefringent on polarized light microscopy
  - o May be invisible on conventional microscopy
  - o Uncommon in malignant lesions
- Type II microcalcifications
  - o Non-crystalline
  - o Calcium, phosphate, hydroxyapatite or phosphorus and calcium with other elements
  - o Found in benign lesions and carcinomas

Clinical Issues

Presentation
- Asymptomatic usually
- Usually screen detected
- Occasionally associated with thickening or lump

Treatment
- No specific treatment
- Routine screening surveillance

Prognosis
- No malignant potential if typical
- Associated heterogeneous calcifications worrisome

Selected References
1. Gunhan-Bilgen I et al: Sclerosing adenosis: Mammographic and ultrasound findings with clinical and histopathological correlation. Eur J Radiol 44:232-8, 2002
2. Frappart L et al: Different types of microcalcifications observed in breast pathology. Correlations with histopathological diagnosis and radiological examination of operative specimens. Virchows Arch A Pathol Anat Histopathol 410:179-87, 1986
3. Sigfusson BF et al: Clustered breast calcifications. Acta Radiol Diagn (Stockh) 24:273-81, 1983

Sclerosing Adenosis

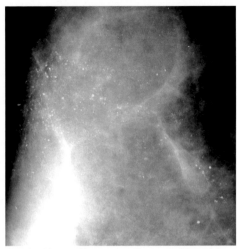

Sclerosing adenosis. 40-year-old asymptomatic woman with suspicious calcifications without similar contralateral findings. Stereotactic vacuum-assisted core biopsy revealed extensive sclerosing adenosis and atypical ductal hyperplasia. Excisional biopsy found florid adenosis without evidence for malignancy.

Key Facts
- Synonym: Adenosis
- Definition: Proliferation of glandular elements
- Classic imaging appearance: Multiple punctate calcifications
- Other Key Facts
  - Benign process
  - Combination of stromal sclerosis and proliferative adenosis
  - Part of the spectrum of fibrocystic change
  - May present a diagnostic challenge for imaging and pathology

Imaging Findings
Mammography Findings
- Nonspecific
- Numerous calcifications
  - Punctate
  - Amorphous
  - Pleomorphic
- Mass
  - Well circumscribed
  - Spiculated
- Architectural distortion
- Asymmetric density

Ultrasound Findings
- Not routinely used to evaluate calcifications
- Masses (palpable and mammographically detected)
  - Non-specific findings
  - Margins well circumscribed – irregular
  - May show posterior acoustic shadowing

MR Findings
- T1 C+: Typically indistinguishable from parenchyma

Sclerosing Adenosis

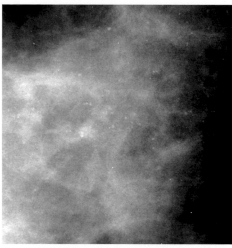

Sclerosing adenosis. 60-year-old asymptomatic woman with a cluster of pleomorphic calcifications in dense breast tissue. Pathology following excisional biopsy revealed sclerosing adenosis with focal atypical lobular hyperplasia.

<u>Imaging Recommendations</u>
- Biopsy recommendation based on imaging characteristic level of suspicion

Differential Diagnosis
<u>Spiculated Malignant Lesions</u>
- Invasive ductal carcinoma, not otherwise specified
- Infiltrating lobular carcinoma
- Tubular carcinoma
  - Helpful to see invasive foci extending beyond adenosis lesion
  - Invasive cells not accompanied by myoepithelial cells
  - Basement membrane absent

<u>In Situ Carcinomas</u>
- May arise in areas of adenosis
- Majority are lobular carcinoma in situ
  - Absence of E-cadherin immunohistochemical activity differentiates from ductal carcinoma in situ

<u>Spiculated Benign Lesions</u>
- Radial scar
  - More extensive sclerosis
  - Central fibrocollagenous scar
- Postoperative scar
  - History usually clarifies imaging findings
  - May be beneficial to mark scar with linear scar marker

Pathology
<u>General</u>
- General Path Comments: Proliferation of lobules and ductules
  - Proliferative adenosis + stromal sclerosis
  - Focal or diffuse
  - Calcifications = 50% lesions

Sclerosing Adenosis

Gross Pathologic, Surgical Features
- Nonspecific findings

Microscopic Features
- Acini elongated and distorted
  - Basement membrane intact
  - Normal two cell layers
- Myoepithelial proliferation
- Stromal fibrosis

Clinical Issues

Presentation
- Typically asymptomatic
- Patient may present with mastalgia
- Less commonly a mass is the presenting finding
  - Adenosis tumor
- Age range 20-67; mean 37-44
- Typically, suspicious imaging findings prompt biopsy

Treatment
- Core biopsy may be adequate
- Excisional biopsy adequate

Prognosis
- Some increased risk (1.7 - 2.5X) for development of invasive carcinoma
- With atypical ductal hyperplasia, risk = 6X

Selected References
1. Gunhan-Bilgen I et al: Sclerosing adenosis: Mammographic and ultrasonographic findings with clinical and histopathological correlation. Europ J Radiology 44:232-8, 2002
2. Cyrlak D, et al. Breast imaging case of the day. RadioGraphics 19:245-7, 1999
3. Bassett LW et al: Diagnosis of Diseases of the Breast. Philadelphia: WB Saunders Co; chapter 25, pp 403-11, 1997

Secretory Calcifications

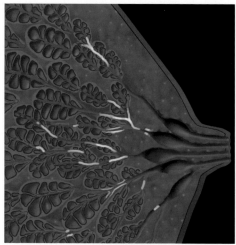

Diagram demonstrates typical secretory calcifications. Dense rod-like calcifications are seen in a ductal distribution with some branching.

Key Facts
- Definition: Benign calcifications in dilated debris-filled ducts, usually composed of calcium phosphate
- Classic imaging appearance: Thick continuous rods > 0.5 mm diameter, with or without lucent centers, may show branching pattern
- Found in
  o Benign secretory changes
  o Plasma cell mastitis (PCM)
  o Mammary duct ectasia (MDE)

Imaging Findings
General Features
- Best imaging clue: Dense, thick, rod-like calcifications in ductal pattern radiating from nipple with occasional branching
- Shape: Rod-shaped with smooth edges typical; may have tapered ends
  o May have some rounded or tubular forms
  o Have been described as "cigar-shaped"
- Size range: 0.5–2 mm diameter
- Location: Any ductal segment
  o Tend to radiate from retroareolar region
Mammography Findings
- Any ductal segment, often bilateral
- Dense, rounded, tubular and rod-shaped calcifications
- Radiate from retroareolar region, may branch
- Sometimes more irregular with prominent branching
  o May be challenging to differentiate from DCIS
Ultrasound Findings
- No specific findings
MR Findings
- No specific findings

Secretory Calcifications

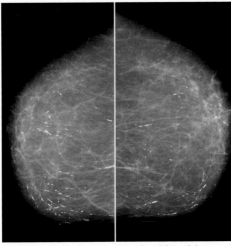

Secretory calcification. CC mammogram views show bilateral dense, rod-like, "cigar-shaped" coarse calcifications some with tapered edges and some showing a branching pattern.

<u>Imaging Recommendations</u>
- Mammography usually characteristic
- No additional imaging required if confident of imaging findings

Differential Diagnosis
<u>Comedocarcinoma</u>
- High nuclear grade DCIS
- Ductal branching pattern of small, fine, linear branching calcifications
- Calcifications may be irregular, "casting" pattern
- Lack lucent centers, smooth margins

Pathology
<u>General</u>
- General Path Comments
  - Lucent centers imply periductal inflammatory changes
- Etiology
  - Dystrophic or degenerative process
  - Intraluminal amorphous debris or secretory material
  - Calcification of debris or material (calcium phosphate)
  - PCM related to prior pregnancy, breast-feeding
  - MDE related to atrophy, phenothiazines, hyperprolactinemia
- Epidemiology
  - PCM usually premenopausal, prior pregnancy & breast-feeding
  - MDE usually postmenopausal, unrelated to parity or breast-feeding

<u>Gross Pathologic, Surgical Features</u>
- Retroareolar dilated ducts
- Ducts may appear thick-walled
- Contain thick, creamy, secretory material

Secretory Calcifications

- Interductal cysts and necrotic areas when severe

Microscopic Features
- Type II calcifications
  - Calcium phosphate mainly, some hydroxyapatite
  - Nonbirefringent under polarized light
- Plasma cell mastitis
  - Ductal epithelial hyperplasia
  - Periductal intense plasma cell infiltrate
  - Intraluminal desquamated epithelium & lipid material
- Mammary duct ectasia
  - Moderate to marked retroareolar duct dilatation
  - Intraluminal debris
    - Amorphous or granular eosinophilic material
    - Lipid-containing foam cells ("colostrum cells")
    - Desquamated epithelial cells
    - Cholesterol crystals and calcifications
  - Periductal inflammation
    - Lymphocytic infiltrate predominant
    - Some plasma cells, neutrophils, histiocytes
    - Fibrosis and hyperelastosis cause duct wall thickening
    - Epithelium atrophic and flattened

Clinical Issues

Presentation
- Most cases asymptomatic, incidental mammographic finding
- Late nipple retraction not uncommon
- Calcifications develop as sequelae to acute phase
- Plasma cell mastitis
  - Younger women (30-45), prior pregnancy
  - Nipple pain, redness and tenderness
  - Thick, creamy discharge common
  - Indurated thickening or mass subacutely
- Mammary duct ectasia
  - Age range 30-80, most 40-70
  - Spontaneous, intermittent nipple discharge
    - Clear, yellow, green, brown
  - No palpable lesion usually
  - Sometimes develop mass (periductal inflammation and fibrosis)

Natural History
- Self-limited
- Tendency for periductal fibrosis and nipple retraction

Treatment
- Rarely needs needle biopsy or surgery to exclude comedocarcinoma
- No specific treatment otherwise

Prognosis
- No malignant potential

Selected References
1. Olson SL et al: Breast calcifications: Analysis of imaging properties. Radiology 169:329-32, 1988
2. Frappart L et al: Different types of microcalcifications observed in breast pathology. Correlations with histopathological diagnosis and radiological examination of operative specimens. Virchows Arch A Pathol Anat Histopathol 410:179-87, 1986
3. Sickles EA: Breast calcifications: Mammographic evaluation. Radiology 160:289-93, 1986

Skin Lesions

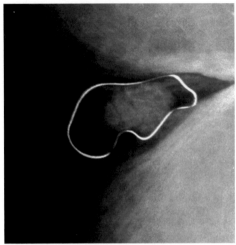

Skin lesion. Raised nevus right axilla in otherwise asymptomatic patient. Magnified MLO view shows that lesion has been appropriately delineated with mole marker.

Key Facts
- Skin lesions often project over breast parenchyma on two-view mammography
  - Most of breast skin superimposed over parenchyma
  - Only small amount of skin is in tangent to x-ray beam
  - Distinguishing skin from parenchymal lesions may be difficult
- Raised lesion should be marked by technologist before exam
  - Small metallic BB or semi-opaque circle marker
    - BB superimposed over lesion most views
    - Lesion identified directly beneath BB on tangential view
- Single or multiple
  - If too numerous, BBs not helpful
- History and visual inspection of the breast essential
  - Meticulous technique to avoid misdiagnosis

Imaging Findings
General Features
- Best imaging clue: Mammographic mass with sharply outlined borders and crevices outlined by air

Mammography Findings
- Shape variable
  - Round
  - Oval
  - Lobulated
  - Irregular
- Margins
  - Usually well-circumscribed

Skin Lesions

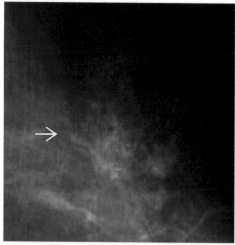

Skin lesion. 76-year-old asymptomatic woman with large seborrheic keratosis over the left upper outer quadrant (arrow). MLO view over unmarked lesion. Note reticular lucencies, representing trapped air, in the crevices of the lesion.

- Small amounts of air trapped by compression at borders produce excellent contrast
- Surface crevices
  - Crenulated surface traps air
    - Fine linear or reticular lucencies
- Calcifications

Ultrasound Findings
- Usually not necessary to make diagnosis

Differential Diagnosis
Seborrheic Keratosis
- Also known as verruca senilis or pigmented papilloma
- Most commonly imaged skin lesion
- Benign
- Greasy feeling to the touch
  - Abundant, fatty, keratinous nest within lesion
- Dark brown, elevated, sharply demarcated
- Mammography
  - Circumscribed, round, oval or lobulated mass
  - May have air in crevices
  - Often see halo around mass from air trapped between border and surrounding skin

Verruca
- Most commonly known as warts
- Represent thickening or projections of epidermis

Benign Nevus
- Shape variable: Round, oval, irregular
- Crevices may be outlined by air
- May develop calcifications

Skin Lesions

- Flat, pigmented skin moles not visible on mammography

<u>Malignant Melanoma</u>
- Usually preceded by flat, hairless mole
  - Not seen on mammography
- Light to dark brown pigment
- Later changes
  - Increase in size
  - Exophytic growth
    - Can be identified on mammography at this point
  - Irregular margins, color variable
- Most common types in breast
  - Superficial spreading
  - Nodular

<u>Epidermal Inclusion Cyst and Sebaceous Cyst</u>
- Clinical and imaging findings indistinguishable
  - Smooth, round, palpable mass
  - Cutaneous or subcutaneous
  - Mammography: Well-circumscribed mass
  - Ultrasound: Usually hypoechoic

<u>Keloid Scar</u>
- May occur after breast biopsy
- Mammography: Irregular, tube-like or mass-like raised structures

<u>Cutaneous Metastases</u>
- Breast, other primary sites

<u>Skin Tags</u>

<u>Mondor's Disease</u>
- Thrombophlebitis of the superficial veins of the breast
- Clinical: Painful, palpable, cordlike structure
  - Mammography: Superficial, tubular density
  - Ultrasound
    - Markedly dilated superficial vessel
    - No flow on Doppler

<u>Neurofibromatosis</u>
- Multiple cutaneous lesions
- Derived from nerve cell sheaths
- Autosomal dominant
- May cover entire body
- Mammography
  - Multiple, bilateral skin lesions
  - Well-defined margins except where lesions attach to skin

Pathology
- Findings pertinent to individual lesions

Clinical Issues
- Findings pertinent to individual lesions/diseases

Selected References
1. Shelty, MK: Mondor's disease of the breast: Sonographic and mammographic findings. AJR 177: 893-96, 2001
2. Bassett LW et al: Diagnosis of diseases of the breast. Philadelphia: WB Saunders Co; Chapter 25, 38-364, 1997
3. Denison, CM: Epidermal inclusion cysts of the breast: Three lesions with calcifications. Radiology. 204:496-96, 1997

Sternalis Muscle

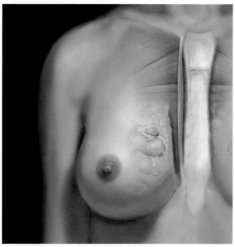

The sternalis muscle can be seen paralleling the right side of the sternum. This muscle has no known function, is present in < 10% of the population, and on mammograms, is visible only on the CC view.

Key Facts
- Definition: A muscle running parallel to the sternum
- Classic imaging appearance
  - Flame-shaped medial density seen only on CC mammogram
- Other key facts
  - < 10% of population
  - Must be differentiated from a focal medial mass

Imaging Findings
Mammography Findings
- Triangular shape
- 1-2 cm in size
- Variable as to irregularity with ill-defined margin
- Medial location adjacent to sternum
- Seen on CC view only
- Cleavage view may be helpful to exclude a true mass
Ultrasound Findings
- Helpful to exclude a mass
CT Findings
- May be helpful in definitive identification
- Medial soft-tissue structure attached to chest wall immediately adjacent to sternum
MR Findings
- T1 C-
  - May be helpful in definitive identification by anatomic location

Differential Diagnosis
Medially-Located Mass
- Benign and malignant masses may develop in medial posterior breast

Sternalis Muscle

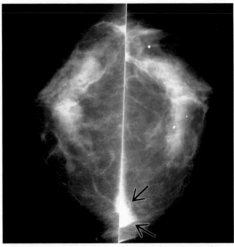

Sternalis muscle. Medial, triangular, somewhat ill-defined density (arrows) seen only on left CC mammographic view represents the sternalis muscle, unilateral in this patient. Prior mammograms showed this finding to be visible and stable for 9 years.

- Careful physical examination and additional imaging studies should discriminate

Variable Attachment of the Pectoralis Muscle
- Small free slip of pectoralis muscle adjacent to sternum
- Visualized on CC view only
  - Round
  - Triangular
  - Flame-shaped
- 1% of women

Pathology
General
- Normal muscle bundle
  - Present in 8% males and females
  - Extends from infraclavicular region to caudal aspect of sternum
  - Unknown function
  - 2/3 unilateral
- Etiology-Pathogenesis
  - Possibly once an extension of rectus abdominus

Clinical Issues
Presentation
- An imaging finding
- Many surveyed surgeons not aware of this finding
Treatment
- None

Selected References
1.   Bailey PM, et al: The sternalis muscle: A normal finding encountered during breast surgery. Plast reconstr surg 103:1189-90, 1999
2.   Kopans D: Breast imaging 2nd edition. Lippincott-Raven, Philadelphia PA; Chapter 2, 9-10, 1998
3.   Bradley FM et al: The Sternalis muscle: An unusual normal finding Seen on mammography. AJR 166:33-6, 1996

Systemic Etiologies

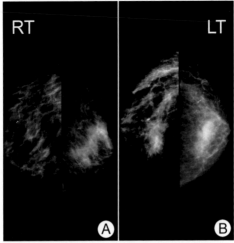

Systemic etiologies. CC and MLO views demonstrate asymmetric findings of edema with trabecular coarsening, overall increased breast density and skin thickening (not visible) more on the right than the left in a 65-year-old woman with hepatic and congestive heart failure. Bilateral vascular calcifications are present.

Key Facts
- Definition: Breast findings associated with systemic disease
  - Collagen vascular disease
  - Vasculitis
  - Athrosclerotic disease
  - Diabetes
  - Renal disease
  - Amyloidosis
  - Steatocystoma multiplex

Imaging Findings
Mammography Findings
- Collagen vascular disease
  - Lymphadenopathy
    - Usually bilateral
    - Rheumatoid arthritis
    - Systemic lupus erythematosus
    - Scleroderma
    - Psoriatic arthritis
  - Dermatomyositis
    - Bizarre, extensive, dystrophic, subcutaneous calcifications
- Vasculitis
  - Wegener's granulomatosis
    - Rarely an irregular or spiculated mass
- Atherosclerotic disease
  - Arterial calcifications
- Diabetes

Systemic Etiologies

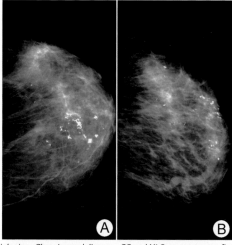

Systemic etiologies. Chronic renal disease. CC and MLO mammogram findings include subcutaneous coarse calcifications and arterial calcifications associated with diffuse findings of edema.

- o Vascular calcifications in younger women
- o Dense breast tissue
  - ▪ May obscure palpable mass(es)
- o Diabetic mastopathy
- Renal disease
  - o Vascular calcifications
  - o Diffuse coarse subcutaneous calcifications
- Associated with secondary hyperparathyroidism
  - o Particularly in dialyzed patients
- Amyloidosis
  - o Dense tissue
  - o Skin thickening
  - o Mass
- Steatocystoma multiplex
  - o Round, well-circumscribed, intradermal masses

<u>Ultrasound Findings</u>
- May be helpful for palpable or mammographically detected masses
- Characteristics nonspecific

<u>Imaging Recommendations</u>
- Mammography may be first examination to suggest systemic disease

Differential Diagnosis

<u>Lymphadenopathy, Bilateral</u>
- Granulomatous diseases
- AIDS
- Mononucleosis
- Leukemia
- Lymphoma

<u>Breast Masses</u>
- Benign and malignant tumors

Systemic Etiologies

Pathology

General

- Breast findings may be disease specific
  - Dermatomyositis
    - Chronic inflammation and degeneration of striated muscle and skin
    - Diagnosis by serum muscle enzyme measurement and muscle biopsy
    - Breast cancer association reported
  - Rheumatoid arthritis
    - When treated with gold, flecks may be present in lymph nodes
  - Scleroderma
    - Skin involvement specific to disease
  - Wegener's
    - Mass may be tender
    - No associated calcifications
    - Biopsy = necrotizing vasculitis of arteries and veins
  - Diabetic mastopathy
  - Amyloid
    - Deposits reported in women with rheumatoid arthritis, multiple myeloma and Waldenström's macroglobulinemia
    - Breast involvement a late development
  - Steatocystoma multiplex
    - Autosomal dominant
    - Uncommon benign cutaneous disorder
    - Intradermal oil cysts
    - Usually in adolescent or young men
- Breast findings may be nonspecific
  - Arteriosclerosis
    - Vascular calcification in younger women may be a predictor of disease
  - Renal disease
    - Edema
    - Calcifications

Clinical Issues

Presentation

- Variable

Treatment

- Disease specific
- Some breast findings may resolve with systemic treatment

Prognosis

- Variable
- Related to disease and comorbid findings

Selected References
1. Shabahang M et al: Surgical management of primary breast sarcoma. Am Surg 68:673-7, 2002
2. Rosen PP: Rosen's breast pathology. Lippincott Williams & Wikins, Philadelphia PA; Chapter 3, 44-58, 2001
3. Feder JM et al: "Unusual breast lesions" radiologic-pathologic correlation. RadioGraphics 19:S11-26, 1999

Tubular Adenoma

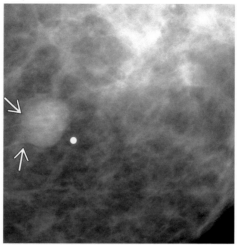

Tubular adenoma. 33-year-old with palpable left breast mass (skin BB over the palpable finding). Mammogram demonstrates an oval mass with one obscured margin (arrows). Surgical excision found a 1.2 cm firm mass; histology = tubular adenoma with surrounding compressed breast tissue.

Key Facts
- Synonym: Pure adenoma
- Definition: Rare benign tumor in young women
- Classic Imaging Appearance
  - Mammographic well-defined mass
  - Sonographic circumscribed hypoechoic mass
- Other key facts
  - Related to fibroadenoma
  - Young women
    - Similar to noncalcified fibroadenomas on mammogram and ultrasound
  - Older women
    - May resemble malignant masses with calcifications

Imaging Findings
Mammography Findings
- Characteristics of fibroadenoma
  - Circumscribed mass
    - Oval
    - Lobulated
    - Round
- Unlike fibroadenoma
  - Tightly packed punctate and irregular microcalcifications
  - No "popcorn" calcifications reported
Ultrasound Findings
- Characteristics similar to fibroadenoma
  - Circumscribed mass
    - Oval
    - Lobulated
    - Round

Tubular Adenoma

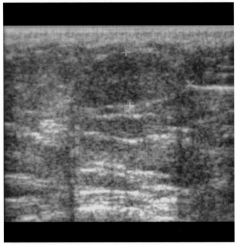

Tubular adenoma. Ultrasound of same case as previous page, shows an oval 1.1 cm, hypoechoic, well-circumscribed mass oriented parallel to the skin with a thin rim, homogeneous internal echogenicity, and slight posterior acoustic enhancement.

- o Homogeneous low level internal echogenicity
- o May have echogenic rim
- May mimic carcinoma

<u>MR Findings</u>
- No reported specific characteristics
- Likely similar to fibroadenoma

Differential Diagnosis
<u>Fibroadenoma</u>
- More common
- Histologic differences
  - o Abundant stroma
  - o Epithelial component of large ducts

<u>Lactating Adenoma</u>
- Pregnant and lactating women
- Prominent tubular and lobular elements with secretory activity

<u>Phyllodes</u>
- Older patients
- Larger lesions
- Cystic spaces within otherwise sonographically similar lesions

Pathology
<u>General</u>
- General Path Comments
  - o Circumscribed mass
  - o Fibroadenoma variant
  - o Other "adenomas" unrelated to fibroadenoma
    - ▪ Apocrine adenoma
    - ▪ Ductal adenoma

Tubular Adenoma

- Pleomorphic adenoma

Gross Pathologic, Surgical Features
- Circumscribed mass
- No true capsule

Microscopic Features
- Closely packed round or oval glandular structures
  - Single layer of epithelium
  - Supported by myoepithelial cells
- Sparse connective tissue
- Microcalcifications may be present
  - Within dilated acinar glands
- Histologic foci may be present within a fibroadenoma

Clinical Issues

Presentation
- Palpable
  - Painless
  - Freely mobile
  - Younger women
- Image detected
  - May have calcifications (not "popcorn-like")
  - > 38 years old

Treatment
- Biopsy recommended for suspicious findings
- Percutaneous core biopsy may provide definitive diagnosis

Prognosis
- Excellent
- No reported increased risk for breast cancer

Selected References
1. Soo MS et al: Tubular adenomas of the breast: Imaging findings with histologic correlation. AJR 174:757-61 2000
2. Rosen PP: Breast Pathology Diagnosis by needle core biopsy. Lippincott Williams & Wikins, Philadelphia PA; chapter 7, 65, 1999
3. Cardenosa G: Breast Imaging Companion. Lippincott-Raven, Philadelphia PA, 252, 1997

Vascular Calcifications

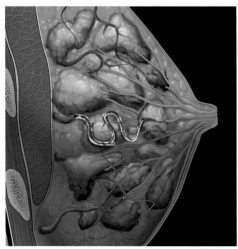

Vascular calcifications. The arteries are pictured as serpiginous branching red structures, the central one of which is partially calcified.

Key Facts
- Synonyms: Breast arterial calcifications (BAC)
- Definition: Calcification within the wall of breast arteries
- Classic imaging appearance
  - Serpiginous pattern of calcifications in a parallel, "tram-track" pattern on mammography
- Other key facts
  - May reflect systemic atherosclerosis
  - May be related to abnormal calcium metabolism
  - May cause large hematoma if unrecognized and biopsied

Imaging Findings
General Features
- Best imaging clue: Serpentine linear and plaque-like calcifications arranged in parallel along vessel wall on mammograms
- Size range: 1-3 mm diameter typically
- Location: Anywhere in breast
Mammography Findings
- Typical calcifications easily recognized
  - Most of single vessel showing mural calcification
  - Calcification in parallel tracks
  - Partly linear, partly plaque-like along vessel wall
  - Tortuous or serpiginous configuration
- Atypical vascular calcifications may mimic malignancy
  - Sometimes limited to short segment
  - Asymmetric calcification along one wall may appear linear, ductal
Ultrasound Findings
- Not usually visible on grayscale US
- May show pulsatile flow on color or power Doppler

Vascular Calcifications

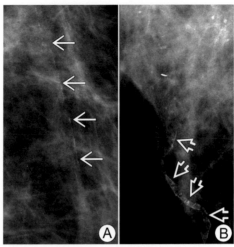

Vascular calcifications. (A) Linear, asymmetric, faint, interrupted, vascular calcifications (arrows) are too elongated for a breast duct; shorter lengths could be confused with ductal calcification. (B) More typical curvilinear vascular calcifications (open arrows) adjacent to multiple benign scattered calcifications.

MR Findings
- Calcifications not visible
- Arteries may be demonstrated on post-contrast scans
- Usually only veins are readily identified

Imaging Recommendations
- Mammographic appearance usually typical
- Magnification views sometimes helpful
- Try to avoid during biopsy of adjacent lesion or suspicious calcifications

Differential Diagnosis
Ductal Carcinoma In Situ
- Linear, often branching calcifications
- Rarely serpiginous, never tortuous
- May have irregular shape, casting configuration
- May show pleomorphic appearance
- Ducts typically arborize more than vessels
  - More branch points in ductal system

Pathology
General
- General Path Comments
  - Calcifications in arterial media (medial sclerosis)
  - Related to systemic atherosclerosis, calcium metabolism disorders
- Etiology-Pathogenesis
  - Reduced in women who have taken hormone replacement therapy (HRT)
  - Common in women on renal dialysis
    - Resolves or reduced after renal transplantation
  - Significant ($p < 0.05$) relationship to various pathological clinical states

- Albuminuria (RR 2.7)
- Hypertension (RR 1.1)
- Transient ischemic attack (TIA)/stroke (RR 1.4)
- Thrombosis (RR 1.5)
- Myocardial infarction (RR 1.8)
- Diabetes for women 65 or older (RR 1.7)
- Epidemiology
  o 8-9% of all screening mammograms
  o 15% of diabetic women
  o Increased frequency with increasing age
  o More common postmenopause
  o Uncommon under 50, even with diabetes

Gross Pathologic, Surgical Features
- No specific features

Microscopic Features
- Calcifications in media of small to medium sized arteries

Clinical Issues

Presentation
- Asymptomatic, screen detected

Treatment
- No specific treatment
- Evaluation for other clinical factors may be useful, esp.
  o Diabetes
  o Renal function and albuminuria
  o Hypertension
  o Previous history of cardiovascular disease

Prognosis
- Often considered clinically insignificant
- Determined by associated clinical factors
- Large scale study shows excess cardiovascular mortality
  o All women: 40% excess (Hazard ratio (HR) 1.4, $p < 0.05$)
  o Diabetic women: 90% excess (HR 1.9, $p < 0.05$)

Selected References

1. Cox J et al: An interesting byproduct of screening: Assessing the effect of HRT on arterial calcification in the female breast. J Med Screen 9:38-9, 2002
2. Kemmeren JM et al: Breast arterial calcifications: Association with diabetes mellitus and cardiovascular mortality. Work in progress. Radiology 201:75-8, 1996
3. van Noord PA et al: Mammograms may convey more than breast cancer risk: Breast arterial calcification and arterio-sclerotic related diseases in women of the DOM cohort. Eur J Cancer Prev 5:483-7, 1996

PocketRadiologist®
Breast
Top 100 Diagnoses

RISK LESIONS

Amorphous Calcifications

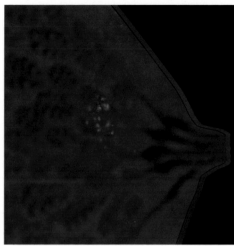

Amorphous calcifications. Diagram shows round, hazy, flake-like, indistinct calcifications. The term "amorphous" is used to describe such calcifications when no other more specific term applies. Cases described as "amorphous" may prove to be benign or malignant on biopsy.

Key Facts
- Definition: Indistinct calcifications that are sufficiently small that a more specific morphologic classification cannot be assigned
- Classic imaging appearance
  - Fuzzy, hazy, round, indistinct, small calcifications
- Lower probability of malignancy than
  - Pleomorphic/heterogeneous/granular calcifications
  - Fine/linear/branching/casting calcifications
- Etiology
  - Benign = 60%
  - Ductal carcinoma in situ = 20%
  - High risk lesions = 20%
    - Atypical ductal hyperplasia
    - Atypical lobular hyperplasia
    - Lobular carcinoma in situ
- Higher rate of malignancy if distribution is
  - Segmental
  - Linear

Imaging Findings
<u>General Features</u>
- Best imaging clue: Small & hazy, round, or "flake" shaped
<u>Mammography Findings</u>
- May be bilateral and in multiple clusters
  - No more likely to be benign than a single cluster
- May identify more with improvement of mammographic technique
- May be stable over multiple years
<u>Ultrasound Findings</u>
- Not identified on US

Amorphous Calcifications

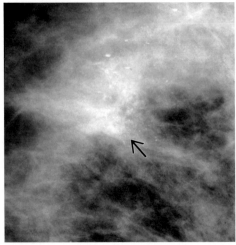

Amorphous calcifications. Mammogram shows faint amorphous calcifications (arrow) representing atypical duct hyperplasia. Note presence of layering milk-of-calcium in association with amorphous forms. Biopsy of most suspicious calcifications should be performed.

<u>Imaging Recommendations</u>
- Magnification views in CC and ML for assessment
  - Findings may show milk-of-calcium
  - One of the mammographic findings that might be labeled as "probably benign"
  - < 2% chance of malignancy = "probably benign"
- Careful attention to any pleomorphic, granular or linear forms
  - Any such abnormal findings should not be followed with imaging
- Biopsy should be performed for any questionable findings

Differential Diagnosis
<u>Atypical Ductal Hyperplasia</u>
- Nonspecific mammographic findings
- Calcifications often prompt biopsy
<u>Atypical Lobular Hyperplasia</u>
<u>Lobular Carcinoma In Situ</u>
<u>Fibrocystic Change</u>
<u>Sclerosing Adenosis</u>

Pathology
<u>General</u>
- General Path Comments; two types of calcifications seen at pathology
  - Calcium phosphate
    - Frequently associated with malignancy
    - Usually found in ducts
    - High density
    - Seen on routine histologic sections
  - Calcium oxalate
    - Frequently associated with benign disease

Amorphous Calcifications

- Usually found in cysts
- Low density, amorphous
- Not clearly visible on routine sections
- Polarized light on microscopy shows calcifications

Gross Pathologic, Surgical Features
- None

Microscopic Features
- Calcifications may be in
  - Ducts
    - Calcium present in the lumen
  - Small cysts
    - Milk-of-calcium

Clinical Issues
Presentation
- No clinical findings

Treatment
- Appropriate to histologic diagnosis

Prognosis
- Excellent if due to benign causes

Selected References
1. Berg WA et al: Biopsy of amorphous breast calcifications: Pathologic outcome and yield at stereotactic biopsy. Radiology 221:495-503, 2001
2. Liberman L et al: The breast imaging reporting and data system; positive predictive value of mammographic features and final assessment categories. AJR 171:35-40, 1998
3. D'Orsi CJ et al. Mammographic feature analysis. Semin Roentgenol 28:204-30, 1993

Architectural Distortion

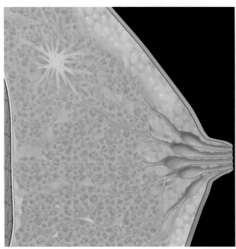

Architectural distortion. Schematic representation of a focal area of distortion. Long spicules are seen as is disruption of the normal fibroglandular contour.

Key Facts
- Definition: Alteration of normal contours of breast parenchyma and stromal elements to produce angular/stellate/spiculated deformity
- Classic imaging appearance
  - Focal angulated deformity of edge of glandular cone
- Other key facts
  - Mammographic sign primarily
  - Surgical scarring most common cause
  - Suspicious but not specific for carcinoma
  - Ultrasonic equivalent: Interruption of stromal lines by shadowing irregular mass or scar
  - MRI equivalent: Spiculated enhancement or distortion around enhancing lesion

Imaging Findings
General Features
- Best imaging clue: Linear opacities radiating from a focal area or point
  - No central mass
  - Focal retraction or distortion of tissue at edge of parenchyma
- Shape: Ill-defined, irregular, spiculated, angulated
- Size range: 5 to 50 mm
- Location
  - Uncommon behind nipple
  - Margins of breast cone typical
  - Axillary tail and upper outer quadrant, especially on MLO
  - Posterior boundary of breast cone, especially on CC view
- Anatomy
  - Cooper's ligaments
    - Arcing curvilinear densities
    - Scalloped concave margins; corresponding shape of adjacent fat

Architectural Distortion

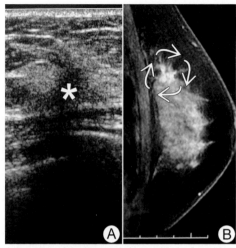

Architectural distortion. (A) Ultrasound shows irregular hypoechoic lesion with interruption of stromal boundaries and posterior shadowing (*). Lesion not found at surgical excision. (B) Post-operative MRI shows spiculated enhancing lesion medial to surgical scar (arrows). Final pathology: Radial scar.

- o Normal glandular cone margins
  - ▪ Convex, curved or smoothly scalloped

Mammography Findings
- "Edge sign": Focal change in margin of glandular cone
  - o Thickening, straightening, angulation with "pulling in"
- "White star" (often carcinoma): Short (< 1 cm) radiating lines, central opacity; may have microcalcifications
- "Black star" (may suggest radial scar): Long (> 1 cm) radiating lines, central fatty lucencies; may have microcalcifications
  - o Nonspecific; may be carcinoma
- Workup views
  - o Required if not postoperative scarring
  - o Confirm distortion is real
  - o Confirm location within breast
  - o Spot compression +/− magnification mandatory
  - o Additional views as required to resolve, confirm or localize
    - ▪ Rolled views
    - ▪ True lateromedial or mediolateral
    - ▪ Stepped oblique views

Ultrasound Findings
- May be normal
- Hypoechoic shadowing mass (lesion) or linear orientation (scar)
- Interruption of stromal architectural lines

MR Findings
- May be normal
- Spiculated enhancement: Strong, moderate or weak enhancement

Imaging Recommendations
- Workup mammographic views if not explained by surgery
- Ultrasound correlation to exclude mass

Architectural Distortion

- MRI if "lesion" not confirmed by imaging or excision

Differential Diagnosis
Normal Overlapping Breast Tissues
- Mimics true architectural distortion
- Resolves with spot compression, no lesion at ultrasound
Surgical Scar, Fat Necrosis
- Correlation with known surgery crucial
- May have dystrophic calcifications
- Becomes less evident with time
Carcinoma
- Spiculations without central mass may be infiltrating cancer
Radial Scar
- "Complex sclerosing lesion" best description
- Often excised for accurate diagnosis
Sclerosing Adenosis
- Benign proliferative process with fibrosis
Focal fibrosis
- Benign perilobular, septal or haphazard fibrotic process

Pathology
General
- General Path Comments
  - Varies with cause of distortion
Gross Pathologic, Surgical Features
- May be normal, no lesion
- Area of focal fibrotic distortion
- Stellate focus or mass
Microscopic Features
- Linear collagenous fibrosis
- Low power shows radiation from central area or lesion
- Central pathology varies with cause

Clinical Issues
Presentation
- Detected incidentally on screening mammogram
- Postoperative surveillance mammogram
- May have palpable thickening or mass
Natural History
- Surgical scar usually resolves at least partially after 1–2 years
- Distortion from scarring worst 6 months post-radiotherapy
Treatment
- Based on lesion histology
Prognosis
- Based on lesion histology

Selected References
1. Pearson KL et al: Efficacy of step-oblique mammography for confirmation and localization of densities seen on only one standard mammographic view. AJR 174:745-52, 2000
2. Krishnamurthy R et al: Mammographic findings after breast conservation therapy. Radiographics 19 Spec No:S53-62, 1999
3. Venta LA et al: Imaging features of focal breast fibrosis: Mammographic-pathologic correlation of noncalcified breast lesions. AJR 73:309-16, 1999

Asymmetric Density

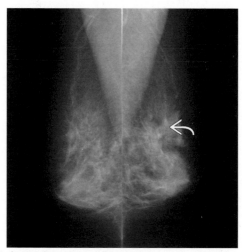

Asymmetric density. Screening mammogram MLO views show an asymmetric density in the left upper breast (arrow). This was not clearly seen on the CC projection.

Key Facts
- Synonym: Asymmetric mammographic density
- Definition: Focal difference in mammographic density of one breast compared to the other; **not** asymmetric breast size
- Classic imaging appearance: Focal increase in mammographic density in one part of one breast; may be seen only in one view
- Other key facts
  - Breast tissue pattern typically fairly symmetrical
    - Minor asymmetry very common
  - Symmetry may fluctuate with physiological factors
    - Aging and glandular involution
    - Hormonal influences especially hormone replacement therapy (HRT)
  - May be technical (positioning, compression, exposure)
  - Usually normal (glandular asymmetry)
  - May be due to benign disease (e.g., stromal fibrosis, cyst)
  - May be due to malignancy (may only be seen on one view)

Imaging Findings
General Features
- Best imaging clue (normal): Visible on only one mammographic view, no focal central density or obvious convex margin
  - May have similar appearance on both mammographic views but lacks borders and the conspicuity of a true mass
- Best imaging clue (mass): Visible on both views, focal central density
Mammography Findings
- Technical asymmetry
  - Characteristically one view only
  - No microcalcifications, architectural distortion, spiculation or true mass
  - Positioning: Difference in position of both breasts in same view

Asymmetric Density

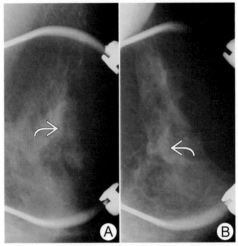

Same patient. Spot compression views in (A) left MLO and (B) left CC projections show vague persistent density with features typical of glandular tissue (arrows). Ultrasound and clinical examination showed normal glandular tissue only.

- o Compression: Under compression causing higher density on one side
- o Exposure: Incorrect positioning of automatic exposure control (AEC) in one view
- Glandular asymmetry, glandular island (most common)
  - o Spreads on spot compression, no central density
  - o No spiculation or distortion
  - o Normal scalloped concave contours
  - o Glandular density intermixed with fat
- True focal lesion
  - o Definable convex margins
  - o Fades into or obscured by surrounding tissue
  - o Usually little or no intermixed fat
  - o Compression and magnification views may reveal
    - Associated distortion, spiculation
    - Microcalcifications
    - Focal lesion margin (e.g., halo, lobulated border)

Ultrasound Findings
- Very high negative predictive value for carcinoma if
  - o Identical to normal glandular parenchyma
  - o No focal palpable abnormality
- Focal ultrasound abnormality
  - o Appearances depend on underlying lesion
  - o Benign, indeterminate or suspicious for cancer

MR Findings
- May be identical to normal glandular tissue
- May show regional moderate enhancement (usually benign)
- May show focal suspiciously enhancing lesion (benign or malignant)

Imaging Recommendations
- Exclude technical asymmetry by analysis of standard views
- Compare with previous films

152

- o Stability, progression, development of new density
- Workup mammography mandatory for true asymmetry
- Ultrasound and clinical examination if focal lesion likely
- Needle biopsy for probable focal mass
- Short-term follow-up of very limited value

Differential Diagnosis
Hormonally Stimulated Glandular Tissue
- Recent use of HRT
Benign Lesion
- Cyst(s)
- Fibroadenoma
- Stromal fibrosis
- Sclerosing adenosis
- Pseudoangiomatous stromal hyperplasia (PASH)
- Infection (e.g., abscess (clinically obvious))
- Granulomatous mastitis
- Papillomatosis
Malignant Lesion
- Invasive ductal carcinoma usually
- Invasive lobular carcinoma notorious; may have some distortion
- Mass-like DCIS occasionally
- Others rare

Pathology
General
- General Path Comments
  - o Findings depend on underlying pathology
- Epidemiology
  - o More common in postmenopausal women
  - o Detectable because of
    - Glandular involution
    - Larger amounts of fat

Clinical Issues
Presentation
- Usually screen detected
- May be symptomatic or clinically detected
  - o Focal thickening or mass
  - o If palpable, further evaluation required
Treatment
- That of underlying pathology
- Routine screening if shown to be glandular asymmetry
Prognosis
- Depends on underlying pathology

Selected References
1. Brenner RJ: Asymmetric densities of the breast: Strategies for imaging evaluation. Semin Roentgenol 36:201-16, 2001
2. Piccoli CW, et al. Developing asymmetric breast tissue. Radiology 211:111-7, 1999
3. Dawson JS, et al. Short-term recall for "probably benign" mammography lesions detected in a three yearly screening program. Clin Radiol 49:391-5, 1994

Atypical Ductal Hyperplasia

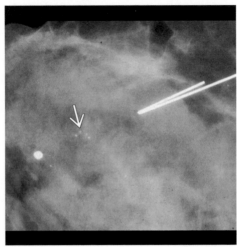

Atypical ductal hyperplasia. Needle localized surgical specimen radiograph demonstrates a cluster of calcifications (arrow) that prompted biopsy in an asymptomatic woman with strong family history of breast cancer. Pathology showed atypical ductal hyperplasia.

Key Facts
- Synonym: ADH
- Definition: Proliferative lesion that fulfills some, but not all, of criteria for ductal carcinoma in situ
- Classic imaging appearance
  - Imaging findings are nonspecific
- Other key facts
  - Considered a high-risk lesion
  - Both breasts at risk
    - When diagnosed on percutaneous biopsy, recommendation should be for surgical excision; ADH may be associated with malignancy
    - May reflect a sampling error with underdiagnosis of malignancy

Imaging Findings
<u>General Features</u>
- Nonspecific mammographic and sonographic findings
- Mammographic findings prompting biopsy
  - Microcalcifications
  - Masses
  - Architectural distortion
  - Asymmetric densities

<u>MR Findings</u>
- Post T1 C+: May have associated neoangiogenesis leading to enhancement patterns similar to malignancy
  - Linear enhancement
  - Focal enhancement
  - Regional enhancement

Atypical Ductal Hyperplasia

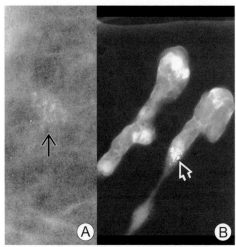

Atypical ductal hyperplasia. (A) 46-year-old asymptomatic woman with a cluster of amorphous calcifications (arrow) sampled with stereotactic vacuum-assisted needle biopsy. (B) Specimen x-ray demonstrated numerous calcifications (open arrow). Core pathology was ADH. Excisional biopsy was negative for malignancy.

Differential Diagnosis
Low-Grade Ductal Carcinoma In Situ (DCIS)
- More ductal areas involved on microscopic assessment
- Both objective and subjective errors may result in under diagnosis of DCIS

Pathology
General
- Some, but not all, cellular features of low-grade DCIS
- Significant variability in pathologists' interpretations
- Area of ductal involvement < 2 mm
  o Despite frank findings consistent with DCIS
- Requires tissue rather than cellular sampling

Microscopic Features
- Structural features of intraductal carcinoma and hyperplasia
- Cribriform or solid architectural ductal cellular arrangement
  o Sharply-defined spaces outlined by distinctly bordered cells
  o Rigid arrangement of cells
- May occur in ducts showing apocrine metaplasia
- Cytologic atypia
  o Nuclear enlargement
  o Distinct cellular borders
  o Easily identified mitotic figures
  o Intracytoplasmic vacuoles may be present

Clinical Issues
Presentation
- May present as a palpable finding
- Biopsy prompted by imaging findings

Atypical Ductal Hyperplasia

Natural History
- May progress to malignancy
  - Not a linear progression

Treatment
- When diagnosed on percutaneous core biopsy
  - Surgical excision should be advised
  - 19-44% of ADH at core biopsy = malignancy at excision
- Following surgical excision
  - Clinical and imaging follow-up

Prognosis
- High-risk lesion for development of breast cancer
  - Both breasts at risk
- Relative risk for developing invasive breast cancer
  - 5x general population
  - 10-11x
    - In woman with concomitant first-degree family history

Selected References
1. Jackman RJ et al: Atypical ductal hyperplasia: Can some lesions be defined as probably benign after stereotactic 11-gauge vacuum-assisted biopsy, eliminating the recommendation for surgical excision? Radiology 224:548-54, 2002
2. Rosen PP: Rosen's breast pathology. Lippincott Williams & Wilkins, Philadelphia PA; Chapter 9, pp 213-5, 2001
3. Page DL et al: Premalignant and malignant disease of the breast; the roles of the pathologist. Mod Patho 11:120-8, 1998

Atypical Lobular Hyperplasia

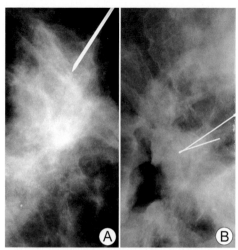

ALH. 60 year old with recent biopsy showing ductal carcinoma in situ with positive margins. Needle-localization re-excision biopsy mammogram (A) shows density and calcifications. Specimen x-ray (B) demonstrates density, architectural distortion and calcifications. Pathology showed extensive ALH with calcifications.

Key Facts
- Synonym: ALH, lobular hyperplastic lesion, lobular neoplasia
- Definition: Atypical epithelium involving lobular units close to but not fulfilling all of the characteristic appearances of lobular carcinoma in situ (LCIS)
- Classic imaging appearance: No specific imaging characteristics
- Other key facts
  - Typically an incidental finding
  - Microcalcifications often prompt biopsy

Imaging Findings
General Features
- Best imaging clue: No specific imaging clues
- Nonspecific mammographic findings
  - Microcalcifications
  - Masses
  - Asymmetric density
  - Architectural distortion
Imaging Recommendations
- Focal suspicious mammographic finding prompts biopsy

Differential Diagnosis
Lobular Carcinoma In Situ (LCIS)
- Qualitative and quantitative histologic differences
Atypical Ductal Hyperplasia
- Differentiation based on cytologic and architectural features
- Not based on site of origin
- ALH may occur in ducts
  - Should be distinguished from duct hyperplasia involving terminal ducts
  - E-cadherin expression is discontinuous, weak, or absent

Atypical Lobular Hyperplasia

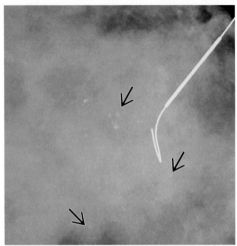

ALH. 60-year-old woman with contralateral ductal carcinoma in situ. Clusters of pleomorphic calcifications (arrows) prompted needle-localization and surgical biopsy with histologic findings of ALH, non-proliferative fibrocystic change, and calcifications associated with benign ducts.

Pathology
General
- There is no uniform histologic definition
- Typically an incidental microscopic finding
- Findings based on quantitative and qualitative findings

Gross Pathologic, Surgical Features
- No specific features

Microscopic Features
- Loss of 2 cell populations above basement membrane
- Near obliteration of lobular lumens in 50% of involved area
- Modest distention of lobules
- Small to moderate clear cytoplasm with rounded nuclei
- Some, but not all, of the features and involvement of LCIS

Clinical Issues
Presentation
- No specific signs
- Palpable mass may prompt biopsy

Treatment
- Following percutaneous biopsy findings of ALH
  - Treatment controversial
  - Literature = 41 of 4332 reported mammotome biopsy cases
    - 24 of 41 (59%) had excisional biopsy
    - 5 of 24 (21%) found carcinoma
  - Our surgeons typically excise ALH found at core biopsy
- Once ALH diagnosed
  - Imaging and clinical follow-up

Prognosis
- Relative risk for developing cancer = 4x controls

Atypical Lobular Hyperplasia

- Risk higher with first-degree family history of breast cancer (= 8x)
- Risk higher with pagetoid spread into ducts

Selected References
1. Dmytrasz K, et al: The significance of atypical lobular hyperplasia at percutaneous breast biopsy. The Breast Journal 9:10-12, 2003
2. Rosen PP: Rosen's breast pathology. Lippincott Williams & Wilkins, Philadelphia PA; Chapter 33, 610-17, 2001
3. Reynolds HE: Core needle biopsy of challenging benign breast conditions: A comprehensive literature review. AJR 174:1245-50, 2000

Axillary Adenopathy

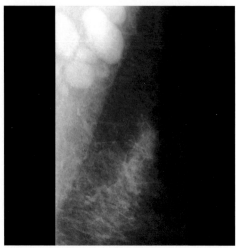

Axillary adenopathy. 39 year old presented with unilateral, large, axillary mass, negative breast exam and negative mammogram. Axillary nodal biopsy = metastatic breast cancer. MRI and ultrasound demonstrated a large upper outer quadrant left breast mass.

Key Facts
- Definition: Pathologic enlargement of axillary lymph nodes
- Classic imaging appearance: Dense nodes with loss of fatty hilum
- 0.3% of mammograms
- Malignant etiologies 55%
- Spread of carcinoma to ipsilateral axilla in breast cancer
  - Prognosis worse & long-term survival decreased
  - Probability of spread correlates with increasing tumor size
- Surgical evaluation necessary in most
  - Sentinel lymph node for prognostic information
  - Axillary dissection for local control

Imaging Findings
General Features
- Best imaging clue: Dense irregular lymph node without fatty hilum
  - The presence of some fat within hilum does not rule out tumor
- Mammography provides limited view of axilla
  - Lower portion of level I nodes seen on MLO view
- Not possible to reliably distinguish malignant from reactive adenopathy
Mammography Findings
- Benign, fatty, hilar infiltration can increase size of normal node to 4 cm
- Loss of fatty hilum (most specific for malignancy)
  - Search for primary tumor in breast
- Extranodal extension can be reliably diagnosed
  - Irregular lymph node margin with spiculation
- Size alone is generally not a strong criterion
  - If > 3 cm, dense, and no fatty hilum, consider suspicious
- Pleomorphic calcifications in node

Axillary Adenopathy

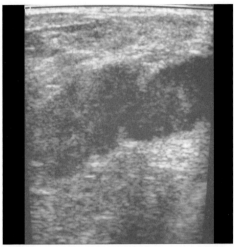

US of metastatic axillary adenopathy shows lobular, irregular, complex mass.

- o Metastatic breast carcinoma
  - Calcifications often similar to primary tumor
- o Metastatic ovarian carcinoma
- Benign, coarse calcifications in node
- o Granulomatous disease
- Gold deposits in node from rheumatoid arthritis treatment

Ultrasound Findings
- Enlarged lymph node with disruption of cortical zone
- May not identify fatty hilum (most specific sign for metastasis)
- May see irregular contour (extranodal extension)

MR Findings
- T1 C+
  - o Does not reliably differentiate between benign & malignant
    - Morphology & kinetics nonspecific
  - o Test of choice for metastatic axillary adenopathy of unknown primary
    - Identifies primary carcinoma in 75-80%
    - May allow breast conservation in lieu of mastectomy

Differential Diagnosis

Primary Breast Carcinoma
- Primary tumor in axillary breast tissue may mimic adenopathy

Unilateral Enlarged Nodes
- Metastatic (breast, melanoma, lung)
- Reactive (inflammation/infection)
- Silicone adenopathy from current or prior rupture

Bilateral Enlarged Nodes
- Benign hyperplasia (Castleman's disease)
- Lymphoma/leukemia
- HIV
- Rheumatoid arthritis/collagen vascular diseases

Axillary Adenopathy

Pathology

General

- General Path Comments
  - o Surgical evaluation is gold standard for suspected metastases
- Anatomy
  - o Level I – lateral to pectoralis minor muscle
  - o Level II – posterior to pectoralis minor muscle (Rotter's nodes)
  - o Level III – medial to pectoralis minor muscle
  - o Average total # nodes: 15–25
- Etiology-Pathogenesis
  - o Malignant cells travel from breast to axilla in stepwise fashion
    - ▪ Level I affected first, followed by II then III
    - ▪ "Skip" metastasis occurs < 5%
- Epidemiology
  - o Probability of axillary metastasis increases with size of primary
    - ▪ Tumor < 1 cm – 20%
    - ▪ Tumor < 2 cm – 33%
    - ▪ Tumor < 3 cm – 45%
    - ▪ Tumor < 4 cm – 50%
    - ▪ Tumor < 5 cm – 60%
    - ▪ Tumor > 5 cm – 70%

Gross Pathologic, Surgical Features

- Nodes are usually visible and palpable in axillary fat

Microscopic Features

- Malignant cells in capsule lymphatic channels & peripheral sinusoids

Staging or Grading Criteria

- Stage II – metastasis to moveable ipsilateral lymph node(s)
- Stage III – metastasis to fixed/matted ipsilateral lymph node(s)
- Stage IIIB – metastasis to ipsilateral internal mammary lymph node(s)

Clinical Issues

Presentation

- Palpable mass under arm

Treatment

- When sentinel node positive, standard approach is full level I & II axillary dissection
- Internal mammary lymph node dissection not standard at most centers
- Axillary radiation
  - o For selected patients at risk for regional nodal failure

Prognosis

- Micrometastasis may adversely affect prognosis
- Poorer overall prognosis
  - o Extracapsular extension
  - o Macroscopic nodal involvement

Selected References
1. Bombardieri E: PET imaging in breast cancer. Q J Nucl Med 45:245-56, 2001
2. Cody HS et al: Complementarity of blue dye and isotope in sentinel node localization for breast cancer: Univariate and multivariate analysis of 966 procedures. Ann Surg Oncol 8:13-9, 2001
3. Walsh R et al: Axillary lymph nodes: Mammographic, pathologic, and clinical correlation. AJR 168:33-8, 1997

Fine Linear Calcifications

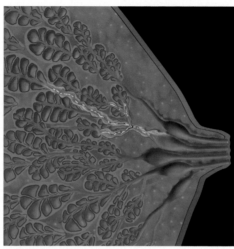

Fine linear calcifications. Diagram depicts calcifications, fine and linear because of their location within small, branching, dilated ducts filled with abnormal cells. The distribution modifier in this case is "linear branching."

Key Facts
- Synonyms: Branching, casting, dot-dash
- Definition: Thin, irregular calcifications that appear linear but are discontinuous, measuring 0.5 mm in width
- Classic imaging appearance
  - Linear branching "Y" or "V"-shaped irregular calcifications
- Appearance suggests filling of the lumen of involved duct irregularly with breast carcinoma (casting)
- High probability of malignancy
  - High-grade (ductal carcinoma in situ) DCIS is likely diagnosis
  - With or without invasion

Imaging Findings
General Features
- Best imaging clue: Linear & irregular, conforming to ductal pattern
Mammography Findings
- Extent of carcinoma may be underestimated on mammography
  - More accurate measurements in high-grade DCIS than low-grade
Ultrasound Findings
- Calcifications may be seen
- May see associated mass
  - Often invasive component
  - Can direct US-guided biopsy
Imaging Recommendations
- Magnification CC & true lateral
- Biopsy indicated
- Post-excision magnification mammography for residual calcifications

Fine Linear Calcifications

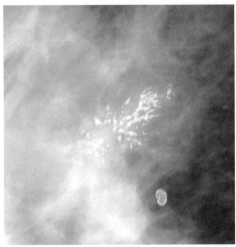

Mammogram of high-grade ductal carcinoma in situ at a lumpectomy site compatible with recurrence.

Differential Diagnosis
Fibroadenoma
- Early calcification in involuting fibroadenoma may mimic carcinoma

Fat Necrosis
- Early calcification can appear malignant

Benign Secretory Disease
- Calcifications typically are coarse, rod-shaped, smooth & tapered
  - Early forms may be worrisome and appear malignant

Pathology
General
- General Path Comments
  - Calcification generally calcium phosphate
- Embryology-Anatomy
  - Ductal carcinoma arises at the junction of terminal duct and lobule terminal duct lobular unit (TDLU)
- Etiology-Pathogenesis
  - Necrotic debris in duct calcifies
  - Linear, branching calcifications more often seen with high-grade DCIS (comedocarcinoma)

Gross Pathologic, Surgical Features
- If comedocarcinoma, will see caseating yellow debris

Microscopic Features
- Solid growth of large cells with poorly-differentiated nuclei
- High mitotic rate generally
- Central necrosis with calcification

Clinical Issues
Presentation
- Typically mammographic finding

Fine Linear Calcifications

Natural History
• High-grade DCIS will invariably progress to invasion

Treatment & Prognosis
• If malignant, surgical excision
• Good, if purely intraductal

Selected References
1. Dershaw DD et al: Patterns of mammographically detected calcifications after breast-conserving therapy associated with tumor recurrence. Cancer 79:1355-61, 1997
2. Holland R et al: Microcalcifications associated with ductal carcinoma in situ: Mammographic-pathologic correlation. Semin Diagn Pathol 11:181-92, 1994
3. Bassett LW: Mammographic analysis of calcifications. Radiol Clin North Am 30:93-105, 1992

Lobular Carcinoma in Situ

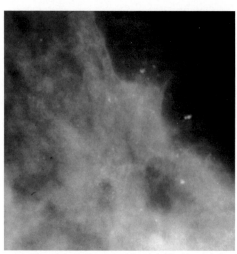

LCIS. 57-year-old woman with contralateral infiltrating lobular carcinoma. Mammographic findings of pleomorphic calcifications and architectural distortion prompted needle localized surgical biopsy. Pathology demonstrated LCIS with the calcifications found in benign ducts and breast stroma.

Key Facts
- Synonyms: LCIS, lobular neoplasia
- Benign high-risk marker for development of invasive carcinoma
  - Both breasts at equal risk to develop invasive cancer
- No classic imaging or clinical characteristics
- Often an incidental pathologic finding
- Frequently bilateral

Imaging Findings
General Features
- No specific mammographic or sonographic findings
- Typical mammographic findings prompting biopsy
  - Calcifications
  - Densities

Differential Diagnosis
Atypical Lobular Hyperplasia (ALH)
- Quantitative and qualitative microscopic differences
Intralobular Extension of Ductal Carcinoma In Situ
- Differentiate with E-cadherin (immunostain)
  - Immunoreactivity absent in LCIS
Proliferative Changes Affecting Terminal Ducts and Lobules
- "Pseudolactational" hyperplasia
- Differentiating microscopic findings
  - Clear cell changes
  - Apocrine metaplasia

Pathology
General
- Expansion of lobules with uniform monomorphic epithelial cells

166

Lobular Carcinoma in Situ

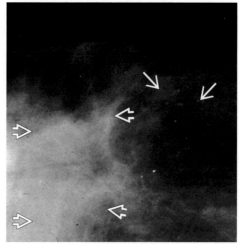

LCIS. 51-year-old asymptomatic woman with mammographic findings of tissue density (open arrows) and pleomorphic calcifications (arrows). Biopsy showed LCIS with calcifications in benign ducts.

   o No myoepithelial cells

Gross Pathologic, Surgical Features
- No specific features

Microscopic Features
- Classic type
  - Small round nuclei
  - No nucleoli
  - Scant cytoplasm
- Pleomorphic type
  - Larger nuclei
    - Some with nucleoli
  - Cytoplasm heterogeneity
    - May contain vacuoles
  - Central necrosis
    - Calcifications may be present

Clinical Issues

Presentation
- No specific signs

Treatment
- Surgical excision following LCIS diagnosed with percutaneous core biopsy
  - Controversial
  - Must demonstrate radiologic/pathologic concordance
  - May be different based on pathologic type of LCIS
  - Recommendations based on a small number of cases
  - Many recommend surgical excision
- Imaging and clinical surveillance following final diagnosis

Prognosis
- Relative risk for developing cancer = 8-11x general population
  - Both breasts at equal risk

Lobular Carcinoma in Situ

- o Invasive cancer may be ductal or lobular
- Relative risk not affected by family history of breast cancer

Selected References
1.   Georgian-Smith D: Calcifications of lobular carcinoma in situ of the breast radiologic-pathologic correlation. AJR 176:1255-9, 2001
2.   Rosen PP: Rosen's breast pathology. Lippincott Williams & Wikins, Philadelphia PA; Chapter 33, 581-610, 2001
3.   Bassett LW et al: Diagnosis of diseases of the breast. Philadelphia: WB Saunders Co; Chapter 25, 429, 1997

Nipple Discharge

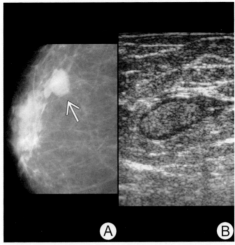

Nipple Discharge. (A) Mammogram of a woman with spontaneous bloody nipple discharge shows well circumscribed uncalcified mass (arrow). (B) US show solid oval mass in a focally dilated duct. Pathology: intraductal papilloma.

Key Facts
- Definition: Secretion from one or multiple ducts
- 99% of all nipple discharge benign
- Classic imaging appearance
  - Filling defect in duct on galactography and/or ultrasound (US)
  - Mammogram usually negative
- Types of nipple discharge
  - Bloody, serous, serosauguinous, watery
    - May be associated with pathology
  - Green – usually indicates fibrocystic disease/duct ectasia
  - White – usually indicates lactation
- Clinically significant pathologic nipple discharge suspected if
  - Unilateral, single duct
  - Bloody, serous, serosauguinous or watery
  - Spontaneous
- 7-10% of clinically significant discharge malignant
  - 50% serous
  - 50% bloody
- Papilloma is most common lesion to cause clinically significant discharge
- Bilateral nonspontaneous non bloody discharge from multiple ducts
  - Is benign
  - May require endocrine evaluation for physiologic cause
- Cytology of nipple discharge
  - False positive 3-4%
  - False negative 12-35%
- Ductal lavage/ductoscopy experimental

Imaging Findings
General Features
- Best imaging clue: Filling defect in duct on galactography and/or US

Nipple Discharge

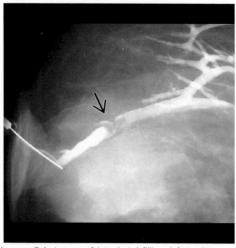

Nipple discharge. Galactogram of intraductal filling defect. Biopsy = intraductal carcinoma in situ.

- Mammography initial evaluation, followed by galactography then US

Mammography Findings
- Usually unrevealing
- Small percentage
  - Linear/branching calcifications
  - Dilated duct
  - Mass

Ultrasound Findings
- Ductal dilation
- Intraductal debris &/or filling defect(s)

MR Findings
- T1 C+
  - Investigational though may be used as adjunctive study

Galactography Findings
- Filling defects
- Duct irregularity/beading/narrowing/distortion/truncation
- Duct usually dilated distal to the lesion

Differential Diagnosis
None

Pathology
General
- General Path Comments
  - Most common lesion identified = papilloma or papillomatosis (40%)
  - Least observed lesion = intraductal carcinoma (5-20%)
- Etiology-Pathogenesis
  - Lactation/pregnancy/post-lactation
  - Fibrocystic disease
  - Intraductal papilloma
  - Duct ectasia

Nipple Discharge

- o Nipple adenoma
- o Infection/chronic mastitis
- o Subareolar abscess
- Epidemiology
  - o Malignancy more likely if
    - ▪ Patient > 50 years
    - ▪ Associated mammographic or US finding
    - ▪ Associated palpable finding
    - ▪ Cytology positive

Clinical Issues
<u>Presentation</u>
- Guaiac may be performed on nipple discharge
- Trigger point may elicit discharge

<u>Treatment</u>
- Any filling defect on galactography should be evaluated pathologically
- 11g vacuum assisted percutaneous biopsy may be used to remove entire lesion with US guidance (controversial)
- Preoperative ductography followed by duct excision
  - o Preoperative ductography technique
    - ▪ 1:1 methylene blue and contrast
    - ▪ Orthogonal galactogram views
  - o Galactographic views may be used to direct needle localization
- Blind surgical duct excision usually eliminates discharge
  - o May not remove responsible lesion

<u>Prognosis</u>
- Depends on underlying lesion

Selected References
1. Slawson SH et al: Ductography: How to and what if? Radiographics 21:133-50, 2001
2. Dennis MA et al: Incidental treatment of nipple discharge caused by benign intraductal papilloma through diagnostic mammotome biopsy. AJR 174:1263-8, 2000
3. Van Zee et al: Preoperative galactography increases the diagnostic yield of major duct excision for nipple discharge. Cancer 82:1874-80, 1998

Papillary Lesions

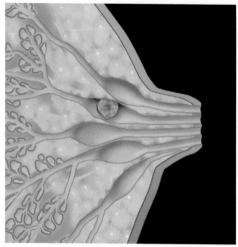

Papillary lesions diagram shows a solitary central uncalcified mass consistent in location and appearance with a solitary benign papilloma.

Key Facts
- Synonyms: Papillary cystadenoma, ductal adenoma, adenomyoepithelioma, intracystic papilloma
- Definition: Discrete tumors of mammary duct epithelium
- < 10% of lesions undergoing breast biopsy
- 1-2% of breast carcinomas
- Papillary neoplasms
  - Benign
  - Malignant papillary carcinomas
- Classic imaging appearance
  - Solitary uncalcified mass or calcifications
- Benign papillomas; solitary more common than multiple
  - Solitary (usually subareolar)
  - Multiple
    - Central
    - Peripheral (more common)
- Differentiate from papillomatosis
  - Microscopic duct hyperplasia

Imaging Findings
General Features
- Best imaging clue: Solitary uncalcified mass or calcifications
Mammography Findings
- Cannot reliably distinguish malignant from benign
- Most common mammographic appearances
  - Solitary uncalcified mass(es) or calcifications
  - Masses with "shell-like" calcifications
  - Asymmetric opacities
  - Dilated ducts
  - Architectural distortion
- Central papillomas

Papillary Lesions

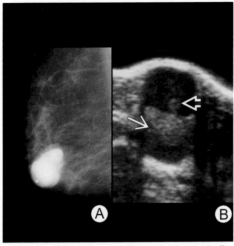

Mammogram = smooth, dense oval mass. Ultrasound with a stand-off pad shows the palpable lesion (elevating the overlying skin) with a dependent fluid-fluid level (arrow) and a small mass (open arrow). Biopsy = intracystic papillary carcinoma with hemorrhage (accounting for appearance of the internal fluid).

- o Usually negative
- o Asymmetrically dilated subareolar ducts
- o Subareolar nodule and/or subareolar amorphous calcifications
- Multiple peripheral papillomas
  - o Round, oval, slightly lobulated, well-circumscribed nodules
  - o Foci of calcifications

Ultrasound Findings
- Cystic component of solid intracystic papilloma may be seen
  - o If not seen, indistinguishable from solid mass

Ductography Findings
- Examination of choice for detecting symptomatic papillomas
- Involved duct usually dilated
- Intraluminal filling defect
  - o May obstruct or distort duct

Imaging Recommendations
- Preoperative ductography may be useful to identify duct
- Needle localization of filling defect may be useful

Differential Diagnosis
Fibroadenoma
Cyst
Intramammary Lymph Node
Papillary/Mucinous/Medullary Carcinoma

Pathology
General
- Papilloma
  - o Localized proliferation of ductal epithelium of ≥ 1 enlarged duct
  - o Proliferation supported by arborized fibrovascular stroma

Papillary Lesions

- Papillary carcinoma
  - Similar to papilloma but has carcinomatous epithelium
- Papillomatosis
  - Papillary hyperplasia involving epithelium of ≥ 1 duct
  - Little or no dilation; sparse supporting fibrovascular stroma
- Papillary DCIS
  - Similar to papillomatosis but has carcinomatous epithelium
- Found within major subareolar or subsegmental duct
  - Multiple peripheral papillomas
- Arise within terminal duct lobular unit
- Associated with atypia, LCIS & radial scars
- Duct dilation not due to obstruction
  - Fluid production exceeds resorption
- Epidemiology
  - Solitary – older 60 yrs
  - Multiple – younger 40-50 yrs

Gross Pathologic, Surgical Features
- Cyst formed by dilated duct in which the papilloma arises can be seen
  - May contain clear or bloody fluid or clotted blood
  - Papilloma usually forms a single mural nodule
- Papilloma may grow as soft friable mass that obliterates cystic space
  - Leads to bloody nipple discharge

Microscopic Features
- Proliferating ductal epithelium on frond-forming fibrovascular stroma
- Presence of apocrine metaplasia or sclerosing adenosis
  - Suggests benign papilloma

Clinical Issues

Presentation
- Solitary central papillomas
  - Nipple discharge (52-100%): Bloody, serous or clear
- Multiple peripheral papillomas
  - Less likely to present with nipple discharge (20%)
  - More likely to present as a palpable or mammographic mass
  - Bilateral more common (14%) than solitary
  - Recurrence after surgery more common (24%)

Natural History
- Multiple peripheral papillomas
  - Increase risk of carcinoma (10-33%)
  - Increase risk of recurrence

Treatment
- Traditional treatment is surgical
  - To differentiate benign from malignant and treat discharge
- Percutaneous core biopsy
  - Usually adequate for diagnosis of benignity (some controversy)

Prognosis
- Based on lesion type

Selected References
1. Rosen EL et al: Imaging-guided core needle biopsy of papillary lesions of the breast. AJR 179:1185-92, 2002
2. Liberman L et al: Percutaneous large-core biopsy of papillary breast lesions. AJR 172:331-7, 1999
3. Cardenosa G et al: Benign papillary neoplasms of the breast: Mammographic findings. Radiology 181:751-5, 1991

Pleomorphic Calcifications

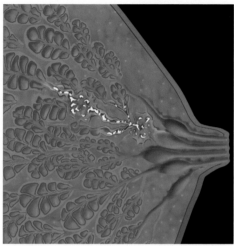

Pleomorphic calcifications. Characteristics of the calcifications include variation in shapes and sizes. The distribution often suggests ductal location. Biopsy findings may be malignant or benign.

Key Facts
- Synonyms: Heterogeneous, granular calcifications (Ca++)
- Definition
  - Irregular calcifications of varying size & shape
  - More conspicuous than amorphous Ca++
  - Neither benign nor typically malignant (linear, linear branching)
  - Usually < 0.5 mm in size
- Classic imaging appearance
  - Small irregular Ca++ of different shapes & sizes
- Other key facts
  - Malignancy probability rate of pleomorphic Ca++ based on distribution
    - Linear 80%
    - Segmental 60%
    - Clustered 40%
    - Regional 40%
  - Overall have an intermediate risk for malignancy

Imaging Findings
<u>General Features</u>
- Best imaging clue: Irregular Ca++ of different size & shape

<u>Mammography Findings</u>
- Ca++ of different size & morphology
- May be clustered, linear or segmentally distributed

<u>Ultrasound Findings</u>
- Ca++ alone usually not seen on US
- May identify associated mass (possible invasive component)

<u>Imaging Recommendations</u>
- Magnification mammography for characterization & distribution
- Biopsy recommended
- If malignant, post-excision magnification to assess residual Ca++

Pleomorphic Calcifications

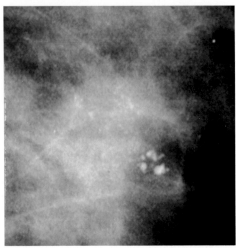

Pleomorphic calcifications. Pathology yielded ductal carcinoma in situ.

Differential Diagnosis

<u>Ductal Carcinoma In Situ (DCIS)</u>
• Subtype can not be predicted based on morphologic pattern of Ca++
<u>Atypical Duct Hyperplasia</u>
<u>Fat Necrosis</u>
<u>Fibroadenoma</u>
<u>Papilloma</u>

Pathology

<u>General</u>
• General Path Comments
   o Pleomorphic Ca++ associated with comedo & noncomedo DCIS
   o Single DCIS lesion can contain both comedo & noncomedo subtypes
      ▪ One subtype generally predominates
   o Comedo DCIS more likely to be associated with
      ▪ Microinvasion
      ▪ Absence of estrogen receptors
      ▪ Over-expression of HER 2/neu oncogene
      ▪ Angiogenesis of surrounding stroma
   o Extent of Ca++ in comedo DCIS correlates well with pathologic size
• Etiology-Pathogenesis
   o Ca++ formed by
      ▪ Necrotic cells that have not yet coalesced to form linear casts (comedo)
      ▪ Calcified secretions in the cribriform spaces (noncomedo)
• Epidemiology
   o Atypia found on percutaneous biopsy requires open excisional biopsy
      ▪ 50% upgraded to DCIS/invasion at surgery (14 gauge)
      ▪ 20% upgraded to DCIS/invasion at surgery (11 gauge)
   o 70–80% of all Ca++ referred for biopsy are benign
   o Pleomorphic Ca++ have an intermediate risk for malignancy

Pleomorphic Calcifications

Microscopic Features
• Ca++ mostly found in ducts

Clinical Issues
Presentation
• No clinical findings
Natural History
• If DCIS, progression to invasion in 33–50% cases
• Unable to prospectively identify lesions that will progress to invasive cancer
Treatment
• None for benign causes
• Mastectomy for > 2.5 cm DCIS
• Breast conservation alone for < 2.5 cm DCIS
  o Recurrence 2-7% per year
    ▪ ~50% invasive carcinoma
• Breast conservation & whole breast radiation therapy for < 2.5 cm DCIS
  o Recurrence lower 1-2% per year
    ▪ ~50% invasive carcinoma
  o Recommended treatment due to lower recurrence rate
Prognosis
• Mastectomy 98% cure rate
• Recurrence rates as above

Selected References
1. Liberman L et al: Breast imaging reporting and data system (BI-RADS). Radiol Clin N Am 40:409-30, 2002
2. Stomper PC et al: Ductal carcinoma in situ: The mammographer's perspective. AJR 162:585-91, 1994
3. Stomper PC et al: Ductal carcinoma in situ of the breast: Correlation between mammographic calcification and tumor subtype. AJR 159:483-5, 1992

Radial Scar

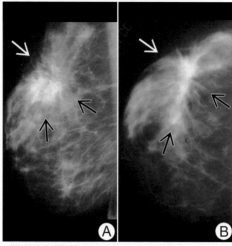

Radial scar. (A) MLO & (B) CC mammogram demonstrates a very large area best characterized as architectural distortion without true central mass. Note the very long spicules. Initial biopsy results of "complex sclerosing lesion" were questioned because of strong concern for cancer. AFIP consultation verified the diagnosis.

Key Facts
- Synonyms: Radial sclerosing lesion (RSL), complex sclerosing lesion, sclerosing duct hyperplasia, non-encapsulated sclerosing lesion
- Definition: Benign proliferative lesion with a spiculated appearance radiographically and histologically
- Classic imaging appearance: Spiculated mass or area of distortion that usually contains central lucency
  - Not specific
  - Same appearance may = invasive carcinoma
- Other key facts:
  - Association with lobular carcinoma in situ (LCIS), ductal carcinoma in situ (DCIS) & tubular carcinoma
  - RSL detected on mammography more likely to be
    - Associated with malignancy (compared to incidental RSL at surgery)
    - Larger (12 mm vs 4 mm)

Imaging Findings
General Features
- Best imaging clue: Architectural distortion with long spiculations radiating from a lucent central point
Mammography Findings
- Variable appearance on different projections
- No central mass (lucency at center)
- May be calcified (33%)
- Long radiating spicules
Ultrasound Findings
- Most mammographically detected RSLs are seen
- Features similar to carcinoma
- Posterior acoustic shadowing may be prominent finding

Radial Scar

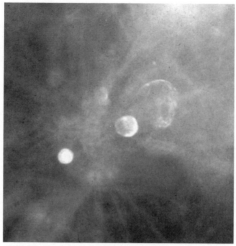

Radial scar. Magnification image demonstrates a vague central density from which long spicules emanate. Benign coarse calcifications, some fat-containing, are associated with the biopsy proven radial scar.

Differential Diagnosis
<u>Tubular Carcinoma</u>
• Indistinguishable radiographically
<u>Infiltrating Carcinoma Not Otherwise Specified (NOS)</u>
• Indistinguishable radiographically

Pathology
<u>General</u>
• General Path Comments
  ○ Similar appearance to small invasive carcinomas on gross
• Etiology-Pathogenesis
  ○ Unknown
  ○ Not related to surgery or prior trauma
• Epidemiology
  ○ Most common 40–60 years
<u>Gross Pathologic, Surgical Features</u>
• Irregular, gray-white & indurated with central retraction
<u>Microscopic Features</u>
• Hypertrophic fibroelastic core
  ○ Surrounded by stellate projections of ducts
    ▪ With varying degrees of hyperplasia
    ▪ Peripheral ducts may be dilated cystically
  ○ Contains trapped glandular elements
    ▪ May be confused with tubular carcinoma
• Various proliferative components in RSL
  ○ Sclerosing adenosis
  ○ Duct hyperplasia
  ○ Cysts

Radial Scar

Clinical Issues
<u>Presentation</u>
- No palpable mass generally

<u>Natural History</u>
- Some increased risk of developing invasive breast carcinoma

<u>Treatment</u>
- When diagnosed on percutaneous biopsy (controversial)
  - o Surgical excision
  - o If no associated atypical ductal hyperplasia (ADH) or (LCIS)
    - Imaging follow-up
  - o Recent report of RSL diagnosed by core biopsy in a screening population: (Suggests that RSL without DCIS, ADH or LCIS may not require surgical excision)
    - RSL at core biopsy led to surgical excision
    - Sensitivity = 85% on stereotactic core biopsy
    - No surgically excised cases associated with invasive cancer
    - Cases with (DCIS) also had the DCIS or atypical ductal hyperplasia in core biopsy specimen

<u>Prognosis</u>
- Good

Selected References
1. Cawson JN: Fourteen-gauge needle core biopsy of mammographically evident radial scars. Is excision necessary? Cancer 97:345-51, 2003
2. Cohen MA et al: Role of sonography in evaluation of radial scars of the breast. AJR 174:1075-8, 2000
3. Jacobs TW et al: Radial scars in benign breast-biopsy specimens and the risk of breast cancer. NEJM 340:430-6, 1999

Skin Thickening and Retraction

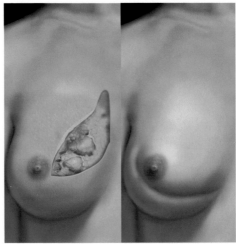

Diagramatic representation of skin thickening (left image) and scarring (right image).

Key Facts

- Definitions
  - Skin thickening: > 2 mm thickness on imaging
  - Skin retraction: Pulling in of skin
- Classic imaging appearance: Retracted or thickened scar may be visible on at least one of 2 standard mammography images
  - May be challenging on film-screen mammography
  - Digital mammography may be optimized to visualize skin
- Seen in benign & malignant conditions
- Skin retraction
  - Focal (most common)
- Skin thickening
  - Diffuse (more common)
- Inflammation, benign and after radiation
- Direct invasion of dermal lymphatics by tumor cells
- Secondary edema due to obstruction by tumor cells
  - Focal (less common)
  - Usually due to post-surgery or infection
  - Late sign of carcinoma

Imaging Findings

General Features
- Best imaging clue: Skin thickness > 2 mm

Mammography Findings
- Skin thickening & retraction often overlooked
  - Tangential view required to detect
- Small areas of skin imaged on mammogram
  - Digital mammography improves evaluation
- Skin retraction
  - Search for underlying carcinoma

Skin Thickening and Retraction

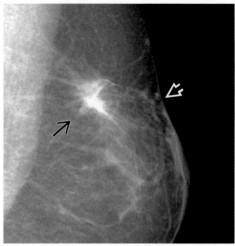

Mammogram of a woman who underwent breast conservation and radiation therapy. The lumpectomy site (arrow) appears as a spiculated scar which causes retraction (open arrow) of the overlying skin.

<u>Ultrasound Findings</u>
- Can directly measure skin thickening; no distinction malignant vs benign
- Verifies clinical impression
- Dilated lymphatics & ducts

<u>T1 C+ MR Findings</u>
- Suspicious for malignancy
  - Thickened skin with enhancement
- Inflammatory carcinoma
  - Suspicious enhancing lesion under area of retraction
- Not suspicious for malignancy
  - Thickened skin without enhancement
- Post-radiation
- Post-biopsy
  - Non-enhancing distortion under area of retraction

Differential Diagnosis

<u>Skin Thickening</u>
- Mastitis
- Nonspecific inflammation
- Neglected carcinoma
- Locally advanced breast carcinoma (LABC)
- Inflammatory carcinoma
  - Shorter clinical symptoms than neglected carcinoma/LABC
- Edema
  - After axillary node dissection
  - Axillary node recurrence
- Systemic diseases
  - Findings typically bilateral
  - Congestive heart failure/anasarca/superior vena cava syndrome/ scleroderma/dermatomyositis/psoriasis

Skin Thickening and Retraction

Skin Retraction
- Scarring from prior biopsy
- Underlying malignancy
- Mondor's disease
- Fat necrosis

Pathology
General
- General Path Comments
  - Breast cancer may extend to skin via
    - Contiguous spread
    - Ductal network and lymphatics
  - Lymphangitic congestion of skin
    - Associated with trabecular thickening
    - Drainage of skin continuous with breast lymphatics
- Embryology-Anatomy
  - Cooper's ligaments attach the breast to the skin
    - Tethering of Cooper's ligaments causes retraction
  - Ductal epithelium in direct continuity with skin
  - Normal skin thickness = 0.5 – 2 mm
    - Except: Inframammary crease, cleavage, periareolar region (thicker)
- Etiology-Pathogenesis
  - Skin thickening
    - Underlying malignancy
    - With inflammatory component
    - Without inflammatory component
  - Post-biopsy
  - Post-radiation
    - Usually diffuse and associated with trabecular thickening
  - Skin retraction
  - Underlying malignancy
    - Desmoplastic reaction to superficial cancer
  - Post-biopsy scarring

Clinical Issues
Presentation
- Skin changes from malignancy are late findings
  - Usually clinically apparent
Natural History
- Post biopsy changes & post-radiation skin thickening
  - Generally self-limiting
Treatment
- None for non-malignant causes
Prognosis
- Good for non-malignant causes

Selected References
1. Gunhan-Bilgen I et al: Inflammatory breast carcinoma: Mammographic, ultrasonographic, clinical, and pathologic findings in 142 cases. Radiology 223:829-38, 2002
2. Kopans DB: Breast imaging. Lippincott Williams & Wikins, Philadelphia PA; chapter 13, 339-43, 1998
3. Harris JR et al: Diseases of the breast. Lippincott Williams & Wikins, Philadelphia PA; chapter 4, 68-9, 1996

PocketRadiologist®
Breast
Top 100 Diagnoses

MALIGNANCIES

Adenoid Cystic Carcinoma

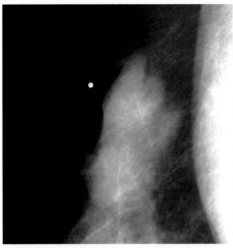

Adenoid cystic carcinoma. Magnified CC view of palpable right upper outer quadrant mass in a 55-year-old woman. Partially-circumscribed, obscured, dumbbell-shaped mass in dense breast tissue. Screening mammogram one week earlier was interpreted as normal.

Key Facts
- Synonym: Cylindroma
- Definition: Rare type of adenocarcinoma
  - Morphologically indistinguishable from adenoid cystic carcinoma of salivary glands
- Classic imaging appearance: Circumscribed, lobulated mass
- Other key facts:
  - Slow growth
  - Mean age = 60
  - < 1% of all breast cancers
  - Very good prognosis

Imaging Findings
General Features
- Size range: 0.2-12 cm
  - Median size 2 cm
- Subareolar most common site
Mammography Findings
- Variable characteristics
  - Circumscribed mass most common
    - Often lobulated
  - Ill-defined mass
  - Focal asymmetric density

Differential Diagnosis
Circumscribed Mass
- Fibroadenoma
- Medullary carcinoma
- Mucinous carcinoma

Adenoid Cystic Carcinoma

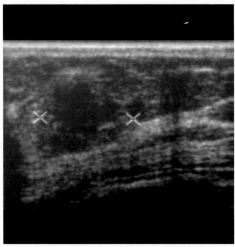

Adenoid cystic carcinoma. Ultrasound of medial aspect of mass demonstrates ill-defined borders, inhomogeneous internal echo-texture, and no acoustic enhancement.

- Metastasis

Ill-Defined Mass
- Infiltrating ductal carcinoma (not otherwise specified)

Pathology

General
- General Path Comments
  - Low incidence of axillary node metastasis
  - Distant metastasis uncommon
    - Lung most common site
  - Most tumors ER/PR negative

Gross Pathologic, Surgical Features
- Gray to pale yellow mass
- Firm
- Circumscribed

Microscopic Features
- Characterized by glandular and stromal elements
- Two main cell components
  - Modified fusiform myoepithelial cells
  - Glandular cuboid cells
- Three structural subtypes
  - Glandular
    - Epithelial cell nests permeated by cylindric spaces
  - Tubular
    - Epithelial strands surrounded by hyaline stroma
  - Solid
    - Solid epithelial strands
- Microscopic invasive growth pattern = 50% of cases

Adenoid Cystic Carcinoma

Clinical Issues

Presentation
- Palpable, tender, subareolar or central mass
  - Not associated with nipple discharge
  - Isolated cases reported in men and children
- No tendency for bilaterality

Treatment
- Best treatment not yet established
- Lumpectomy followed by radiation therapy insufficiently studied
- Mastectomy most common surgical treatment
- Adjuvant chemotherapy not yet evaluated

Prognosis
- Excellent

Selected References
1. Arpino G et al: Adenoid cystic carcinoma of the breast: Molecular markers, treatment and clinical outcome. Cancer 94(8):2119-27, 2002
2. McClenathan JH: Adenoid cystic breast cancer. Am J Surg 183:646-9, 2002
3. Santamaria G et al: Adenoid cystic carcinoma of the breast: Mammographic appearance and pathologic correlation. AJR 171:1679-83, 1998

DCIS - General

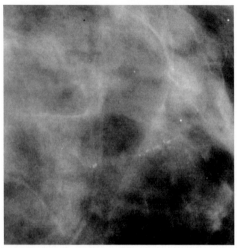

Ductal carcinoma in situ. Mammogram of fine, linear, branching calcifications that suggest filling of the lumen of a duct.

Key Facts
- Synonyms: Ductal carcinoma in situ (DCIS), preinvasive, noninvasive or intraductal cancer
- Definition: Clonal proliferation of epithelial cells originating in terminal duct lobular unit with intact basement membrane
- 20–40% of all breast cancers diagnosed by mammography
- Microcalcifications = cardinal finding
- Multifocality
  - DCIS in multiple sites in 1 quadrant
- Multicentricity
  - DCIS in > 1 quadrant
  - More frequent in lesions > 2–2.5 cm

Imaging Findings
<u>Mammography Findings</u>
- Classic appearance
  - Calcifications 80%
    - Develop secondary to tumor necrosis
    - May develop secondary to secretions
  - Typical calcification morphology
    - Granular, pleomorphic, casting
    - Pleomorphic
    - Casting
  - Typical calcification distribution
    - Linear, linear-branching, clustered
  - Mass with associated calcifications = 10%
  - Mass = 10%
- Not able to predict grade based on pattern of calcification
<u>Ultrasound Findings</u>
- Usually not detected though may be visible
  - Microlobulated mass

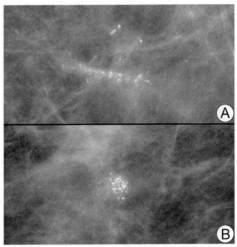

Ductal carcinoma in situ. (A) Mammogram of fine, linear and granular calcifications in a linear distribution. (B) Mammogram of cancerization of the lobule where ductal carcinoma in situ has extended retrograde into the lobule.

- Mild hypoechogenicity
- Ductal extension
- Normal acoustic transmission
  o Dilated duct with hypoechoic nondependent echoes

MR Findings
- T1 C+
  o Linear or ductal clumped enhancement most common
  o Mass enhancement less common
  o Kinetic curves not reliable

Imaging Recommendations
- Biopsy of any suspicious calcifications, regardless of stability
- Preoperative assessment of extent of tumoral calcifications
  o Routine use of magnification orthogonal views
  o Entire breast should be examined for multicentricity
- Specimen radiography should be routinely used
- Postoperative mammogram within several weeks if breast conserved
  o Assess for residual suspicious calcifications
- Follow-up mammogram at 6 months for new baseline
  o Typically at time of radiation therapy treatment completion

Differential Diagnosis
Atypical Duct Hyperplasia
- Quantitative and qualitative microscopic differences
Sclerosing Adenosis
- Proliferative lobulocentric lesion derived from the terminal lobular unit

Pathology
General
- Pathologic classification of DCIS evolving
- Three types based on nuclear pleomorphism

- o Low
- o Intermediate
- o High nuclear grade
- Two types based on architecture
  - o Comedocarcinoma
    - ▪ Associated with necrosis & casting calcifications
  - o Noncomedocarcinoma
    - ▪ Solid, papillary, micropapillary, cribriform
- Embryology-Anatomy
  - o Arises in terminal ductal lobular unit (TDLU) and grows in duct toward nipple
    - ▪ Continuous (comedo)
    - ▪ Discontinuous (noncomedo) pattern
  - o Cancerization of the lobule: DCIS grows retrograde into lobule
- Epidemiology
  - o Diagnosed more frequently due to mammographic screening
    - ▪ Prior to more extensive mammography use = 5% of mammography-detected breast cancer
    - ▪ With increased mammography use = 20-40%

Staging or Grading Criteria
- Stage 0

Clinical Issues
Presentation
- Asymptomatic in majority
- Symptomatic
  - o Mass
  - o Spontaneous nipple discharge
  - o Paget's disease

Natural History
- Relationship of DCIS to invasive cancer controversial
- DCIS may persist for years before becoming invasive
- Risk of developing into invasive cancer
  - o Low grade = lowest risk
  - o High grade = highest risk

Treatment
- Lumpectomy with negative margins
- Mastectomy may be recommended
  - o Multicentric or > 2.5 cm DCIS
  - o Extensive high-grade DCIS
- Radiation therapy following lumpectomy based on size and nuclear grade
- Tamoxifen for estrogen receptor (ER+)

Prognosis
- High cure rate if adequately treated

Selected References
1. Rosen PP: Breast pathology. Lippincott-Raven. 209-74, 1997
2. Lagios MD et al: Mammographically detected duct carcinoma in situ: Frequency of local recurrence following tylectomy and prognostic effect of nuclear grade on local recurrence. Cancer 63:618-24, 1989
3. Stomper PC et al: Clinically occult ductal carcinoma in situ detected with mammography: Analysis of 100 cases with radiologic-pathologic correlation. Radiology 172:235-41, 1989

DCIS - High Grade

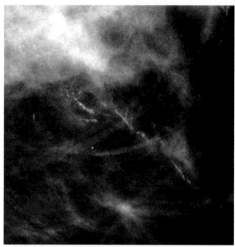

DCIS – high grade. Mammogram of linear, branching, casting calcifications in a linear distribution. The appearance suggests filling of the lumen of a duct involved irregularly by breast cancer.

Key Facts
- Synonyms: Poorly differentiated ductal carcinoma in situ, high-grade DCIS, comedocarcinoma
- Definition: Pathologic classification indicating high aggressiveness
- Linear branching calcifications on mammography
- Mammography fairly accurate in estimating lesion size

Imaging Findings
<u>General Features</u>
- Calcifications = hallmark
  - Classic exuberant linear & branching calcifications
  - Other morphologies
    - Granular, irregular, heterogeneous, pleomorphic
  - Distribution reflects duct or ductal segment
- Most likely DCIS sub-type to be associated with calcifications
- Mammography can more reliably estimate size of lesion
- A mass may be associated with calcifications
  - Suspicious for invasive component
- Alternate imaging may be helpful to assess noncalcified high grade DCIS
<u>Ultrasound Findings</u>
- Dense casting calcifications may be seen
  - Biopsy with US may be possible
- No particular features
- Generalized hypoechoic irregular tissue
<u>T1 C+ MR Findings</u>
- Clumped linear or ductal enhancement in majority
- Mass enhancement less common
- Kinetic curves not reliable
- No more likely to exhibit enhancement than low or intermediate grades

DCIS - High Grade

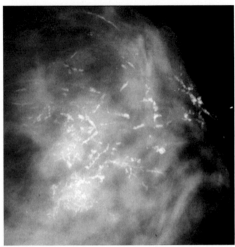

DCIS- high grade. Mammogram of linear, branching, casting calcifications in a segmental distribution in the immediate subareolar position.

Imaging Recommendations
- Preoperative assessment of extent of tumoral calcifications
  - o Routine use of orthogonal magnification views
  - o Maximal extent of the calcifications should be reported
  - o Entire breast should be examined for multicentricity
- Mammogram can fairly reliably estimate lesion size
  - o More so in this sub-type than in intermediate or low-grade DCIS
- Specimen radiography should be routinely used
- Postoperative mammogram within several weeks if breast conserved
  - o Assess for residual suspicious calcifications
    - ▪ Routine and magnification views
- Follow up mammogram at 6 months for new baseline
  - o Typically at time of radiation therapy treatment completion

Differential Diagnosis
Low and Intermediate-Grade DCIS
- Calcification morphology and distribution not specific
  - o Cannot reliably differentiate histologic findings of DCIS sub-types
Atypical Duct Hyperplasia
- Quantitative and qualitative microscopic differences
Sclerosing Adenosis
- Proliferative lobulocentric lesion
- Derived from the terminal ductal lobular unit (TDLU)

Pathology
General
- General Path Comments
  - o Pathologic classification of DCIS evolving
  - o Classification by grade based mainly on nuclear cytology
  - o Presence or absence of necrosis & architecture can be considered

DCIS - High Grade

- Comedocarcinoma usually high grade
- Papillary & micropapillary infrequently high grade
- Cribriform rarely high grade
- Comedocarcinoma is a gross descriptive term
  - DCIS that has areas of necrosis that calcify
- Epidemiology
  - Diagnosed more frequently now because of mammographic screening

Gross Pathologic, Surgical Features
- Extensive comedo type of DCIS shows visible tissue abnormality
  - Granular character with pale yellow foci of necrotic debris
  - Necrotic material exudes from the ducts

Microscopic Features
- Tumor cells have high nuclear grade & extensive necrosis
- Comedo architecture primarily
- Mitotic figures

Staging Criteria
- Stage 0

Clinical Issues

Presentation
- Asymptomatic in majority
- Calcifications on mammography most common
- Palpable mass

Natural History
- Majority of high-grade DCIS progresses to invasion

Treatment
- Lumpectomy – wide local excision with negative margins
- Radiation therapy
- Mastectomy may be recommended
  - Multicentric
  - Extensive high grade DCIS
- Tamoxifen for estrogen receptor-positive tumors
- Sentinel lymph node biopsy (controversial)

Prognosis
- Excellent cure rate if adequately treated
- Most likely type of DCIS to recur
  - Recurrence rates differ
    - Mastectomy vs lumpectomy
    - With and without radiation therapy
  - If there is recurrence, > 50% invasive
- Lower favorable prognosis
  - High nuclear grade
    - More important than architectural growth pattern
  - Necrosis
  - Positive surgical margin, large lesion size

Selected References
1. Moon WK et al: Multifocal, multicentric, and contralateral breast cancers: Bilateral whole-breast US in the preoperative evaluation of patients. Radiology 224(2):569-76, 2002
2. Holland et al: Ductal carcinoma in situ: A proposal for a new classification. Semin Diagn Pathol 11:167-80, 1994
3. Holland et al: Extent, distribution and mammographic/histological correlations of breast ductal carcinoma in situ. Lancet 335:519-22, 1990

DCIS - Intermediate Grade

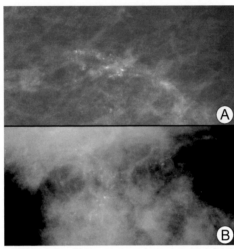

DCIS - intermediate grade. (A) Mammogram shows segmental distribution of fine granular calcifications. (B) Mammogram shows regional distribution of pleomorphic calcifications.

Key Facts
- Synonyms: Intermediate grade DCIS, non-comedocarcinoma
- Definition: Pathologic classification indicating intermediate aggressiveness
- Classic mammographic appearance
  - Calcifications
  - Calcifications may be present in only part of the DCIS

Imaging Findings
Mammography Findings
- Best imaging clue: Microcalcifications
  - Granular
  - Delicate, fine, irregular
  - Pleomorphic
  - May be monomorphic
Ultrasound Findings
- Usually negative
- Less likely to see calcifications than with high-grade DCIS
MR Findings
- T1 C+
  - Linear or ductal clumped enhancement in majority
  - May appear as irregular mass though less common
  - Kinetic curves not reliable
Imaging Recommendations
- Biopsy of any suspicious calcifications, regardless of stability
  - DCIS may be present for years before progressing to invasion
- Preoperative assessment of extent of tumoral calcifications
  - Routine use of orthogonal magnification views
  - Maximal span of the calcifications should be reported
  - Entire breast should be examined for multicentricity

DCIS - Intermediate Grade

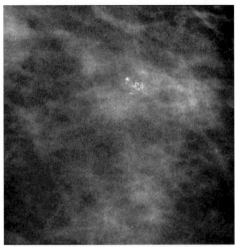

DCIS - intermediate grade spot magnification view shows a cluster of pleomorphic calcifications. Biopsy revealed intermediate grade DCIS.

- Mammogram may underestimate extent of DCIS
  - Low- and intermediate-grade DCIS extent underestimated by 2 cm
    - 50% of cases
  - Underestimation more likely with increasing lesion size
- Specimen radiography should be routinely used
  - To confirm sampling of calcifications
- Postoperative mammogram within several weeks if breast conserved
  - Assess for residual suspicious calcifications
    - Routine and magnification views
- Follow-up mammogram at 6 months for new baseline

Differential Diagnosis
High-Grade and Low-Grade DCIS
- Calcification morphology and distribution not specific
  - Cannot reliably differentiate histologic findings of DCIS sub-types
Atypical Duct Hyperplasia
- Quantitative and qualitative microscopic differences
Sclerosing Adenosis
- Proliferative lobulocentric lesion
- Derived from the terminal ductal lobular unit (TDLU)

Pathology
General
- General Path Comments
  - Pathologic classification of DCIS evolving
  - Considered intermediate grade
    - Cribriform, solid or papillary pattern & no necrosis
    - Cribriform, solid or papillary & necrosis
    - Lacks nuclear anaplasia of comedocarcinoma
- Micropapillary subtype more often associated with
  - Nipple discharge

- o Paget's disease
- o Palpable mass
- o Multicentric disease
- Embryology-Anatomy
  - o Arises in TDLU
  - o Grows in duct toward nipple in a discontinuous (noncomedo) pattern
- Epidemiology
  - o Diagnosed more frequently due to mammographic screening

Gross Pathologic, Surgical Features
- None

Microscopic Features
- Intermediate nuclear grade with focal or absent necrosis
- Noncomedo architecture
  - o Often a mixture

Staging Criteria
- Stage 0

Clinical Issues
Presentation
- Asymptomatic in majority
- Calcifications on mammography most common
- Palpable breast lump rare: Micropapillary most common
- Paget's disease or nipple discharge

Natural History
- Data suggest DCIS is precursor lesion
  - o All invasive ductal carcinomas arise from DCIS
  - o DCIS progresses to invasive cancer in 30-50%
- DCIS may persist for years before becoming invasive

Treatment & Prognosis
- Lumpectomy – wide local excision with negative margins
- Radiation may be used
  - o Lesion size
  - o Surgeon/oncologist choice
- Mastectomy
  - o > 2.5 cm DCIS
  - o Multicentric
- Sentinel lymph node biopsy not performed
- Tamoxifen for Estrogen Receptor (ER+)
  - o Decreases risk of developing subsequent invasive cancer
- Excellent cure rate if adequately treated
- Lower favorable prognosis in
  - o Positive surgical margin
  - o Large lesion size

Selected References
1. Jaffer S et al: Histologic classification of ductal carcinoma in situ. Microsc Res Tech 59:92-101, 2002
2. Morrow M et al: Standard for the management of ductal carcinoma in situ of the breast (DCIS). CA Cancer J Clin 52(5):256-76, 2002
3. Goldstein NS et al: Differences in the pathologic features of ductal carcinoma in situ of the breast based on patient age. Cancer 88(11):2553-60, 2000

DCIS - Low Grade

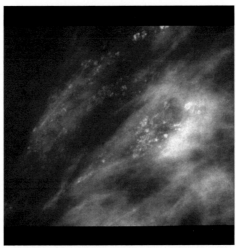

DCIS – low grade. Mammogram reveals regional granular calcifications.

Key Facts
- Synonyms: Low nuclear grade DCIS, well-differentiated DCIS, non-comedocarcinoma
- Definition: Pathologic classification indicating low aggressiveness
- Classic imaging appearance
  - Calcifications
  - Mammographic calcification patterns not helpful predicting tumor grade
- Histologic extent of tumor underestimated by extent of mammographic calcifications

Imaging Findings
Mammography Findings
- Calcifications
  - Develop in secretions
  - Round
  - Punctate
  - Pleomorphic
  - Clustered distribution
Ultrasound Findings
- Usually negative
- Less likely to see calcifications than with high-grade DCIS
T1 C+ MR Findings
- Linear or ductal clumped enhancement most common
- Mass enhancement less common
- Kinetic curves not reliable
Imaging Recommendations
- Biopsy of any suspicious calcifications, regardless of stability
- DCIS may be present for years before progressing to invasion
- Pre-operative assessment of extent of tumoral calcifications
- Routine use of orthogonal magnification views
- Maximal span of the calcifications should be reported

DCIS - Low Grade

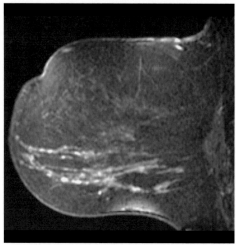

DCIS- low grade. T1 C+ fat suppressed MR image reveals segmental linear clumped enhancement extending from the nipple to the chest wall.

- o Entire breast should be examined for multicentricity
- Mammogram may underestimate extent of DCIS
  - o Low- and intermediate-grade DCIS extent underestimated by 2 cm
    - ▪ 50% of cases
  - o Underestimation more likely with increasing lesion size
- Specimen radiography should be routinely used
- Post-operative mammogram within several weeks if breast conserved
  - o Assess for residual suspicious calcifications
    - ▪ Routine and magnification views
- Follow-up mammogram at 6 months for new baseline

Differential Diagnosis
<u>High and Intermediate-Grade DCIS</u>
- Calcification morphology and distribution not specific
  - o Cannot reliably differentiate histologic findings of DCIS sub-types
<u>Atypical Duct Hyperplasia</u>
- Quantitative and qualitative microscopic differences
<u>Sclerosing Adenosis</u>
- Proliferative lobulocentric lesion
- Derived from the terminal ductal lobular unit (TDLU)

Pathology
<u>General</u>
- General Path Comments
  - o Pathologic classification of DCIS evolving
  - o Any pattern of growth composed of uniform cells
    - ▪ Without atypia
    - ▪ Without necrosis
  - o Lesion classified on basis of highest grade present
- Embryology-Anatomy

- o Arises in TDLU and grows in duct toward nipple in a discontinuous (noncomedo) pattern
- Epidemiology
  - o Diagnosed more frequently due to mammographic screening

Microscopic Features
- Low nuclear grade cells with absent necrosis
- Noncomedo architecture
  - o Solid
  - o Cribriform
  - o Papillary
  - o Micropapillary

Staging Criteria
- Stage 0

Clinical Issues

Presentation
- Asymptomatic in majority
- Calcifications on mammography most common
- Palpable breast lump rare
  - o Micropapillary most common
- Paget's disease or nipple discharge

Natural History
- If left untreated will likely progress to invasive carcinoma
  - o Less aggressive than high grade
  - o Can progress after decades in situ

Treatment
- Lumpectomy – wide local excision with negative margins
- Radiation may be added
  - o Lesion size
  - o Surgeon/oncologist choice
- Mastectomy
  - o Multicentric
  - o > 2.5 cm DCIS
- Tamoxifen for estrogen receptor (ER+)
  - o Decreases risk of developing subsequent invasive cancer

Prognosis
- Excellent cure rate if adequately treated
- Lower recurrence rate compared with high grade

Selected References
1. Ernster VL et al: Detection of ductal carcinoma in situ in women undergoing screening mammography. J Natl Cancer Inst 94(20):1546-54, 2002
2. Verkooijen HM et al: Management of women with ductal carcinoma in situ of the breast: A population-based study. Ann Oncol 13(8):1236-45, 2002
3. Scott MA et al: Ductal carcinoma in situ of the breast: Reproducibility of histological subtype analysis. Hum Pathol 28:967-73, 1997

Infiltrating Ductal CA, NOS

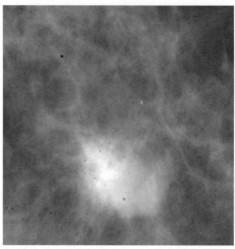

Infiltrating ductal carcinoma, not otherwise specified (NOS). Spot magnification mammogram shows an oval spiculated dense mass without associated calcifications. Biopsy = infiltrating ductal carcinoma NOS.

Key Facts
- Synonyms: Infiltrating ductal carcinoma not otherwise specified (NOS), invasive ductal carcinoma, scirrhous carcinoma
- Definition of invasion: Extension of tumor cells through duct basement membrane
- Definition of NOS: When carcinoma does not fit any defined subtype
- 65% of all breast cancers
- Invasive ductal carcinoma classification
  - NOS 75%
  - Medullary 10%
  - Colloid/mucinous 5%
  - Tubular 5%
  - Papillary 5%
  - Adenoid cystic < 1%
  - Other

Imaging Findings
General Features
- Best imaging clue: Irregular mass
Mammography Findings
- Classic imaging appearance
  - Mass, spiculated and irregular margins = 70%
  - Pleomorphic malignant calcifications
  - Focal asymmetry
  - Architectural distortion
- Higher attenuation than parenchyma 50%
- Less common presentations
  - Diffuse spiculation/reticulation with or without skin thickening
  - Asymmetry or generalized increased density
  - Thickening of Cooper's ligaments

Infiltrating Ductal CA, NOS

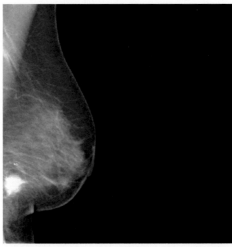

Infiltrating ductal carcinoma NOS. Mammogram of an irregular dense mass in the posterior breast.

  o Skin/nipple retraction
- Other important features
  o Change from a previous mammogram
    ▪ New density; new mass/calcifications
    ▪ Enlarging mass

Ultrasound Findings
- Classic US appearance
  o Irregular hypoechoic shadowing mass
  o Heterogeneous echotexture
  o Taller than wide
  o Thick echogenic rim
- Other appearances
  o Lobulated
  o Homogeneous echotexture
  o Posterior acoustic enhancement

MR Findings
- T1 C+
  o Classic MR appearance
    ▪ Rim-enhancing, spiculated, heterogeneous mass

Differential Diagnosis
Invasive Lobular Carcinoma
Radial Scar
Abscess
Fat Necrosis
Scar
Desmoid Tumor
Metastasis

Infiltrating Ductal CA, NOS

Pathology
<u>General</u>
- General Path Comments
  - o May be associated with abundant fibrosis, desmoplasia & cicatrization
- Genetics
  - o Demographic, reproductive history, family history
  - o Atypia, lobular carcinoma in situ
  - o Radiation exposure
- Embryology-Anatomy
  - o Arises in terminal duct lobular unit

<u>Gross Pathologic, Surgical Features</u>
- Gritty, hard mass

<u>Microscopic Features</u>
- If no distinct features – classified as NOS

<u>Staging or Grading Criteria (If indicated)</u>
- Staging applies to largest mass if > 1 present
- Stage I – tumor < 2 cm
- Stage II – tumor 2–5 cm or positive axillary nodes
- Stage III – tumor > 5 cm or matted nodes
  - o IIIB – skin or chest wall involvement
- Stage IV – metastatic disease

Clinical Issues
<u>Presentation</u>
- Hard palpable mass
- Nipple and/or skin retraction

<u>Natural History, if Untreated</u>
- Vascular and lymphatic invasion
- Skin erosion, ulceration and inflammatory changes possible

<u>Treatment</u>
- Chemotherapy for lymph node involvement or cancer > 1 cm
- Mastectomy
  - o Large tumor
  - o Multicentric (> 1 quadrant) disease
- Breast conservation therapy
  - o Tumor < 5 cm if cosmesis preserved
  - o Unifocal or multifocal (1 quadrant) disease
- Radiation therapy: 4800 rads to breast, 1200 boost to lumpectomy site

<u>Prognosis: 5 Year Survival</u>
- Stage I - 90%
- Stage II - 70%
- Stage III - 50%
- Stage IV - 20%

Selected References
1. Kopans DB: Breast imaging. Lippincott-Raven 576-82, 1998
2. Rosen PP: Breast pathology. Lippincott-Raven 209-74, 1997
3. Harris JR et al: Diseases of the breast. Lippincott-Raven 393-444, 1996

Inflammatory Breast Cancer

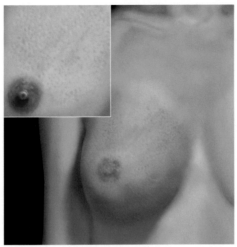

Drawing demonstrates constellation of findings of erythema, skin edema and peau d' orange better appreciated in picture insert.

Key Facts
- Definition: Clinical presentation of rapid onset of diffuse breast changes with aggressive tumor invasion of dermal lymphatics
  - Erythema
  - Warmth
  - Skin edema
  - Dermal ridging (peau d'orange)
- Other key facts
  - May be misdiagnosed as benign inflammatory process
  - < 1% of breast cancers
  - An invasion of dermal lymphatics by aggressive infiltrating tumor
    - Associated mass or malignant calcifications not typical

Imaging Findings
Mammography Findings
- Common features
  - Skin thickening
  - Diffuse increased in breast density
- Other findings may be present
  - Trabecular thickening
  - Axillary lymphadenopathy
  - Architectural distortion
  - Focal asymmetric density
  - Nipple retraction
- Less common features
  - Malignant-appearing calcifications
  - Masses
Ultrasound Findings
- Nonspecific

Inflammatory Breast Cancer

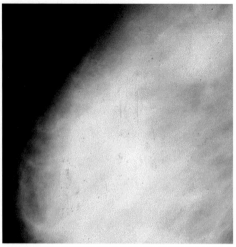

Mammogram demonstrates skin thickening, trabecular thickening and overall increased breast density in a patient with recent onset of erythema, skin changes, warmth and pain throughout the breast.

- o Widening of dermal-subcutaneous fat interface
- o Edematous changes are indistinguishable from tumor infiltration
- May identify mammographically occult mass
- Useful in differentiating inflammatory processes
  - o Focal abscess

MRI Findings
- Little indication for MRI imaging
- T1 C+
  - o Intense rapid enhancement
    - ▪ Typically poorly defined regional or diffuse

Differential Diagnosis
Locally Advanced Breast Cancer With Secondary Dermal Lymphatic Invasion
- Probably a separate entity
- Progression of an infiltrating carcinoma
- Breast masses and malignant-appearing calcifications more common
- Slightly better overall 5 year survival

Benign Inflammatory Process
- Typically in lactating women
- Treatment based on clinical findings
  - o Systemic antibiotics
  - o Abscess drainage
  - o Surgical excision of non-responsive/recurrent abscesses

Pathology
General
- General Path Comments
  - o Age distribution similar to infiltrating ductal carcinoma
    - ▪ Average age 55 years
  - o Skin biopsy may be diagnostic

Inflammatory Breast Cancer

- ▪ May be negative

Gross Pathologic, Surgical Features
- Breast skin changes
  - o Erythema
  - o Thickening
  - o Peau d'orange
  - o Palpable mass uncommon

Microscopic Features
- Diffuse infiltration without well-defined tumor mass
- Infiltrating duct carcinoma
  - o Poorly differentiated
  - o Estrogen-receptor negative
  - o HER 2/neu overexpression
- Intralymphatic dermal tumor emboli
  - o Tumor emboli may be present throughout the breast

Staging or Grading Criteria
- Stage IIIB

Clinical Issues

Presentation
- Breast complaints
  - o Erythema
  - o Warmth
  - o Skin thickening
  - o Peau d'orange
  - o Pain
  - o Mass

Treatment
- Multimodality
  - o Intensive chemotherapy
  - o Mastectomy
  - o Radiation therapy

Prognosis
- Best in cases with good clinical and pathologic treatment response
- Multimodality treatment
  - o 5-year survival up to 50%
- Without multimodality treatment
  - o 5-year survival < 5%

Selected References
1. Rosen PP: Rosen's breast pathology. Lippincott Williams & Wikins, Philadelphia PA. Chapter 35, 676-83, 2001
2. Kushwaha AC: Primary inflammatory carcinoma of the breast: Retrospective review of mammographic findings. AJR 174:535-48, 2000
3. Kopans D: Breast imaging 2nd edition. Lippincott-Raven, Philadelphia PA. Chapter 5, 103, 1998

Interval Cancers

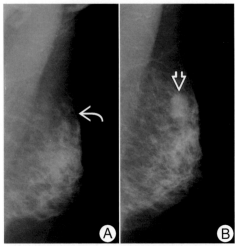

Interval cancers. Left MLO mammograms of a patient taken in August (A) and November (B) of the same year, showing rapid interval development of a focal irregular mass (open arrow), which had become palpable since the mammogram. The equivalent area in the original mammogram (A) marked with (curved arrow).

Key Facts
- Definition
  - Malignant tumors presenting clinically during interval between routine screenings
  - Prior screening study and/or recall assessment did not find cancer
  - Excludes cancers found at next screening round
  - Missed cancer: Overlooked at screening, visible on review
  - True interval cancer: Not visible or not suspicious on review
- Classic imaging appearance
  - May be suspicious but overlooked at prospective initial reading ("missed")
    - Small, poorly-defined, asymmetric density or mass
    - Subtle microcalcifications
    - Subtle architectural distortion
  - May have no suspicious findings on prospective reading ("true interval")
- Other key facts
  - More common in
    - Women under 50
    - Women with very dense breasts (odds ratio (OR) 6.1)
    - Women with previous recall and benign assessment (OR 3.2)
    - Improperly positioned mammograms (OR 2.6)
  - Probably more aggressive than screen-detected cancers

Imaging Findings
General Features
- Best imaging clue: Suspicious clinical findings in woman with a recently reported normal screening study
Mammography Findings
- Typical malignant features often evident at presentation

Interval Cancers

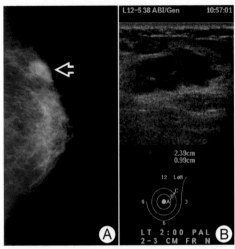

Interval cancers. Same patient, (A) Left CC view shows new irregular mass in lateral breast (arrow) (B) US of palpable lesion shows hypoechoic irregular 2.3 cm suspicious mass. Histology showed an invasive ductal carcinoma with a large number of mitoses and high nuclear grade, consistent with an aggressive tumor.

- Interval cancer classification on retrospective review
  - Missed cancer (visible, suspicious, but not recalled)
    - 15-41% (consensus)
    - 20-38% (single blinded reader)
    - True interval cancer (occult or visible non-suspicious finding), 60-85% (methodology varies)
    - Usually small, poorly-defined density or mass
- Improperly positioned mammograms increase risk (OR 2.6)
- Features with high sensitivity for subsequent interval carcinoma
  - Suspicious microcalcifications (sensitivity 97%)
  - Architectural distortion/stellate (sensitivity 81%)
  - Asymmetric focal density (sensitivity 77%)

Ultrasound Findings
- Ultrasonically suspicious mass usually visible at presentation
- Misclassification of mass on prior ultrasound may occur

Imaging Recommendations
- Careful review of previous imaging
- Short-term follow-up does not reduce interval cancer rate
- Cannot eliminate regardless of screen modality, but may minimize with
  - Quality assurance, positioning crucial
  - Dual reading for screening mammograms (not presently standard of care)
  - Better radiologist training and education
  - Computer aided detection (CAD) may be helpful, but not proven to reduce rate
- Increased recall rate uneconomic
  - Estimated additional 100-400 recalls per interval cancer detected

Interval Cancers

Differential Diagnosis
None

Pathology
General
- General Path Comments
  - Usually higher stage than screen detected cancers
  - More rapid growth, more aggressive than screen-detected cancers
- Genetics
  - No specific genetic factors known
- Etiology-Pathogenesis
  - No specific factors known
- Epidemiology
  - Incidence increases with time after screening
    - First year 2-6 per 10,000 screens
    - 2nd & 3rd years ~10-18 per 10,000 screens
  - More common in
    - Women under 50 (59% of interval cancers in first year)
    - Women with very dense breasts (OR 6.1 compared with fatty breasts)
    - Women with prior benign recall assessment (OR 2.2-3.2)

Microscopic Features
- Typical features of malignancy
- Varies with histological subtype
- Compared to screen-detected cancers
  - More Grade 1 (missed cancers) and Grade 3 (true interval cancers)
  - Much higher proportion of proliferating cells (OR 4.1)
  - More likely to express p53 on immunohistochemical stains (OR 3)

Staging or Grading Criteria
- True interval cancers (compared with screen-detected cancers)
  - Higher incidence of Stage II or greater
  - Median mitotic activity higher ($p < 0.0001$)
  - Larger S-phase fractions ($p = 0.01$)
  - May have higher biological aggressiveness
- Missed cancers similar to screen-detected cancers

Clinical Issues
Presentation
- Usually palpable new lump

Natural History
- No long term survival data

Prognosis
- Screen-detected (missed) cancers may have improved survival as compared with true interval cancers

Selected References
1. Warren RM et al: Radiology review of the UKCCCR breast screening frequency trial: Potential improvements in sensitivity and lead time of radiological signs. Clin Radiol 58:128-32, 2003
2. Gilliland FD et al: Biologic characteristics of interval and screen-detected breast cancers. J Natl Cancer Inst 92:743-9, 2000
3. Mandelson MT et al: Breast density as a predictor of mammographic detection: Comparison of interval-and screen-detected cancers. J Natl Cancer Inst 92:1081-7, 2000

Invasive Lobular Carcinoma

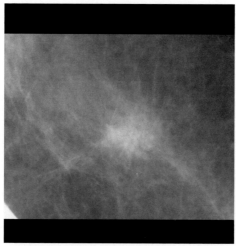

Invasive lobular carcinoma. Mammogram shows spiculated mass.

Key Facts
- Synonyms: Infiltrating lobular carcinoma (ILC)
- Definition: Cytologic features of cells suggest they arose from lobule
- 10% of all breast cancers
- Difficult to detect mammographically due to insidious growth pattern
  - Larger at diagnosis than other cancers
  - May present as palpable mass or thickening
- Accounts for a large number of malpractice suits for diagnosis failure

Imaging Findings
Mammography Findings
- Spiculated high-density mass (most common)
- Asymmetric density without definable margins
- Architectural distortion
- Calcifications rare
- Indistinguishable appearance from infiltrating ductal carcinoma
- More likely to be isodense or hypodense to fibroglandular tissue
- More likely to be seen only on one view (CC most commonly)
Ultrasound Findings
- Vague area of shadowing without defined borders
- Indistinguishable appearance from infiltrating ductal carcinoma
T1 C+ MR Findings
- Indistinguishable from infiltrating ductal carcinoma
- Can be a cause of false negative MR examination
Imaging Recommendations
- MR imaging useful for
  - Disease extent in ipsilateral breast
  - Screening of contralateral breast

Differential Diagnosis
Infiltrating Ductal Carcinoma
- Large crossover in appearances

Invasive Lobular Carcinoma

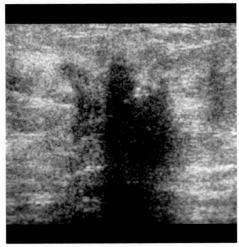

Invasive lobular carcinoma. US shows irregular hypoechoic mass with posterior acoustic shadowing.

Pathology

General
- General Path Comments
  - Growth pattern "single file" of cells that infiltrate breast
    - Results in subtle changes of architecture/density
    - Does not incite intense desmoplastic response
- Etiology-Pathogenesis
  - Exact relationship between lobular carcinoma in situ (LCIS) and ILC unclear
- Epidemiology
  - Occurs at all ages

Gross Pathologic, Surgical Features
- Firm hard tumor with irregular borders
- Usually have a fibrotic, scirrhous appearance
  - Margin may blend in with surrounding parenchyma
- Specimen may not be visibly abnormal in some cases

Microscopic Features
- Variants
  - Classical
    - Slender strands of small cells (1-2 thick) with uniform nuclei infiltrating fibrous stroma
    - Mild to moderately cellular
  - Solid (cellular) pattern
    - Cells arranged as sheets or large, irregularly-shaped nests
  - Alveolar pattern
    - Cells arranged in circumscribed globular nests
    - Nests simulate distended terminal ductules of LCIS
  - Pleomorphic cell type
    - Cells are larger & more atypical than classical
  - Signet-ring cell type
    - Disagreement if solely variant of lobular carcinoma

Invasive Lobular Carcinoma

- o Histiocytoid cell type
  - ▪ Tumor cells have prominent foamy/granular cytoplasm
- o Tubulolobular carcinoma
  - ▪ Small tubules grow in targetoid pattern in a background of classic invasive lobular carcinoma
- o Mixed
- Lymphocytic reaction rare

<u>Staging or Grading Criteria</u>
- Identical to infiltrating ductal carcinoma

Clinical Issues
<u>Presentation</u>
- May be palpable with negative mammogram & US
- More likely to present as interval cancer than other types
- May present with a decrease in affected breast size

<u>Natural History</u>
- Reported higher incidence of
  - o Bilaterality (controversial)
  - o Multicentricity
- Metastasizes frequently to bone, peritoneum, adrenals, gastrointestinal tract, ovary and leptomeninges

<u>Treatment</u>
- Identical to infiltrating ductal carcinoma

<u>Prognosis</u>
- Stage for stage equal to that of invasive ductal carcinoma NOS
- Classic pattern may have a better prognosis
- Solid pattern may have a worse prognosis
- Pleomorphic cell type has poor prognosis
- Tubulolobular carcinoma reported to have
  - o Lower incidence of positive nodes
  - o Lower recurrence rate
  - o Fewer distant metastases
  - o Better overall survival

Selected References
1. Hilleren DJ et al: Invasive lobular carcinoma: Mammographic findings in a 10-year experience. Radiology 178:149-154, 1992
2. LeGal M et al: Mammographic features of 455 invasive lobular carcinomas. Radiology 185:705-708, 1992
3. Sickles EA et al: Subtle & atypical mammographic features of invasive lobular carcinoma. Radiology 178:25-26, 1991

Invasive Papillary Carcinoma

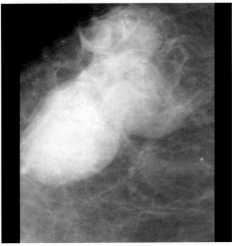

Mammogram of invasive papillary carcinoma shows a lobulated mass containing pleomorphic calcifications.

Key Facts

- Synonyms: Infiltrating papillary carcinoma, intracystic papillary carcinoma with invasion
- Definition: Rare form of specified invasive ductal carcinoma
- Classic imaging appearance: Well-circumscribed mass in elderly patient
- Two types
  - Solid – has higher tendency to invade
  - Cystic – may develop in a dilated lobule or duct
- Aspiration may yield bloody fluid
  - Fluid results from cyst and papillary growth
  - Hemorrhage may occur spontaneously
- Rare, 1-2% of all breast cancers
- May be solitary or multiple
- Not aggressively infiltrative

Imaging Findings

Mammography Findings
- Round, oval or lobulated, fairly well-circumscribed mass
- Multiple masses may occur, often within one quadrant
- Calcifications, if present, are fine and granular
- Spiculation rare as does not produce profuse fibrotic reaction
- Pneumocystography may identify mural mass/irregularity

Ultrasound Findings
- Homogeneously solid or complex solid and cystic mass or masses
- Posterior acoustic enhancement or normal sound transmission
- Intracystic mass or mural nodules
- Papillary projections and septae
- Sequelae of hemorrhage may be seen

MR Findings
- T1 C+
  - Heterogeneous, enhancing, well-circumscribed mass if solid

Invasive Papillary Carcinoma

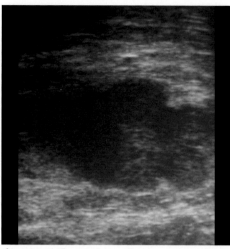

Ultrasound of invasive papillary carcinoma shows a complex cystic structure with a mural mass.

    o Mural/nodular enhancement of cystic mass (±hemorrhage)

<u>Galactography Findings</u>
- May be helpful in evaluation of nipple discharge
- Ductal obstruction, wall irregularity, filling defects seen
- Cannot distinguish between papillary carcinoma with or without invasion

Differential Diagnosis: Circumscribed Breast Masses
<u>Cyst</u>
<u>Fibroadenoma</u>
<u>Hematoma, Infection, Abscess</u>
<u>Papilloma</u>
<u>Phyllodes Tumor</u>
<u>Papillary Ductal Carcinoma In Situ</u>
- May present as single or multiple circumscribed masses
- Similar mammographic and US findings
<u>Invasive Ductal Carcinoma NOS</u>
<u>Invasive Ductal Carcinoma Specified (Medullary or Mucinous, Colloid)</u>
<u>Lymphoma</u>
<u>Metastatic Disease</u>

Pathology
<u>General</u>
- General Path Comments
  - o Hallmark of all papillary tumors (benign or malignant)
    - Proliferating epithelium in villous-like projections fill duct lumen
- Etiology-Pathogenesis
  - o Thought not to arise from solitary papillomas found in large ducts
  - o Unclear whether continuum with peripheral small duct papillomas
- Epidemiology
  - o Older non-Caucasian women
  - o Mean age 65 years

Invasive Papillary Carcinoma

  o Slow growth rate

Gross Pathologic, Surgical Features
- Well circumscribed
- Often contain hemorrhage and cystic areas

Microscopic Features
- Absent myoepithelial layer distinguishes from benign papillary lesion
- Usually not associated with necrosis or calcifications
- Invasive elements are usually at lesion periphery

Staging or Grading Criteria
- Staging identical to invasive ductal carcinoma NOS

Clinical Issues
Presentation
- Firm but not hard, mobile mass
- Mass may be large owing to cystic component
- Nipple discharge in up to one third

Natural History
- Size of invasive component small in relation to lesion size
- Axillary metastases infrequent

Treatment
- Surgical excision with lymph node biopsy/dissection

Prognosis
- Favorable
- 5-yr survival 90%

Selected References
1. Liberman L et al: Case 35: Intracystic papillary carcinoma with invasion. Radiology 219:781-4, 2001
2. Soo MS et al: Papillary carcinoma of the breast: Imaging findings. AJR 164:321-6, 1995
3. Mitnick JS et al: Invasive papillary carcinoma of the breast: Mammographic appearance. Radiology 177:803-6, 1990

Locally Advanced Breast Cancer

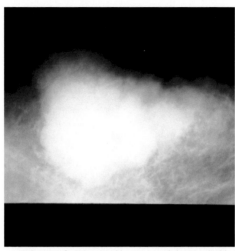

Mammogram. MLO view of a 48-year-old woman with huge palpable breast mass and palpable axillary adenopathy compatible with locally advanced breast cancer. Pathology: High-grade infiltrating ductal carcinoma with lymphatic tumor emboli and extranodal extension of axillary nodes.

Key Facts
- Synonyms: LABC, advanced loco-regional breast cancer, advanced primary breast cancer
- Definition: Historically applied to inoperable disease
  - Defined many different ways
  - Large primary tumors greater than 5 cm (T3)
  - Skin/chest wall involvement (T4) and/or fixed axillary (N2) or ipsilateral internal mammary (N3) lymph node involvement
  - Stage IIIa (T0-2N2 or T3N1-2) and stage IIIb (T4Nx or TxN3) disease
  - Inflammatory breast cancer (IBC) (T4d) is a part of LABC but reported separately
    - Distinct clinical behavior and very poor prognosis
- Clinical features for inoperable breast cancer
  - Extensive edema of skin of breast
  - Satellite nodules in skin
  - Parasternal tumor
  - Inflammatory carcinoma
  - Arm edema
  - Supraclavicular metastases
  - 2 or more of the following
    - Skin ulceration
    - Limited edema of skin of breast
    - Fixation to chest wall
    - Fixation of axillary lymph nodes
    - Axillary nodes > 2.5 cm on palpation
- Classic imaging appearance
  - Diffuse changes on mammogram
    - Density, distortion, mass and/or calcifications

Locally Advanced Breast Cancer

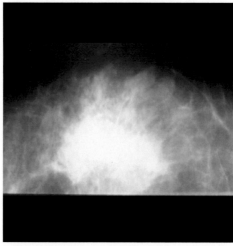

Mammogram. Craniocaudad view of inoperable breast cancer. 51-year-old presented with fixed hard breast mass that invaded pectoralis major muscle but not chest wall. Pathology: Infiltrating ductal carcinoma that responded to chemotherapy.

Imaging Findings

General Features
- Best imaging clue: Large area of parenchymal density or distortion

Mammography Findings
- Large dominant mass
- Large area of suspicious calcifications
- Diffuse increased density
- Large area of architectural distortion
- Skin thickening
- Clinical findings may be more prominent than mammographic findings

Ultrasound Findings
- Large solid irregular mass
- May have diffuse shadowing without discernable mass borders

T1 C+ MR Findings
- Useful for evaluation of
  - Tumor extent
    - Pectoralis major muscle
    - Chest wall (intercostal muscles, ribs, serratus anterior muscle)
    - Skin & nipple
  - Response to chemotherapy

Imaging Recommendations
- Imaging helpful in evaluation of response to chemotherapy
  - Multi-modality approach best (clinical examination, mammography, US, MRI)
  - No modality presently can predict absence of residual disease

Differential Diagnosis

Mastitis
Abscess

Locally Advanced Breast Cancer

Pathology
General
- General Path Comments
  - Infiltrating ductal poorly differentiated
  - If inflammatory component present
    - Much worse prognosis
    - Tumor cells identified in skin lymphatics
- Epidemiology
  - 5% breast cancer in industrialized countries with screening programs
  - 70% breast cancers in developing countries without screening

Clinical Issues
Presentation
- Easily palpable
- May present with diffuse infiltration of breast without dominant mass

Treatment
- Combined modality therapy
- Systemic chemotherapy for inoperable LABC & IBC
  - Provides valuable information about tumor responsiveness
    - Ineffective treatment switched
  - Tumor shrinkage ("down-staging")
    - May allow breast conservation
  - Followed by regional therapy
    - Surgery, radiation therapy
- Hormonal therapy
  - Estrogen receptor (ER) positive tumors
  - Lower recurrence rate than preoperative chemotherapy
- Contraindications for neoadjuvant therapy
  - Multiple operable tumors requiring mastectomy
  - Tumors where response is slow or difficult to assess
    - Invasive mucinous carcinoma
    - Invasive lobular carcinoma

Prognosis
- Depends on response to chemotherapy
  - Complete response – good prognosis
  - Disease progression – extremely poor prognosis
- Evaluation of response can be difficult due to fibrosis or small volume residual disease
  - Multi-modality approach appropriate

Selected References
1. Huber S et al: Locally advanced breast carcinoma: Evaluation of mammography in the prediction of residual disease after induction chemotherapy. Anticancer Res20:553-8, 2000
2. Herrada J et al: Relative value of physical examination, mammography, and breast sonography in evaluating the size of the primary tumor and regional lymph node metastases in women receiving neoadjuvant chemotherapy for locally advanced breast carcinoma. Clin Cancer Res 3:1565-9, 1997
3. Helvie MA et al: Locally advanced breast carcinoma: Accuracy of mammography versus clinical examination in the prediction of residual disease after chemotherapy. Radiology 198:327-32, 1996

Medullary Carcinoma

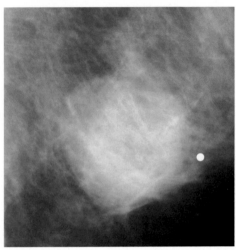

Medullary carcinoma. 43-year-old woman with palpable 9 o'clock left breast lump. Magnified MLO view reveals partially circumscribed round mass. Note indistinct anterior and inferior margins.

Key Facts
- Synonyms: Circumscribed carcinoma, bulky adenocarcinoma, cystic neomammary carcinoma
- Definition: Well-circumscribed carcinoma with poorly-differentiated cells, little stroma, and lymphoid infiltration
- Classic imaging appearance
  - Oval or lobulated circumscribed mass on mammogram
- Other key facts
  - < 5% of all breast cancers
  - Rapid growth
  - Mean age 46-54
  - Locally aggressive

Imaging Findings
Mammography Findings
- Typical type
  - Oval lobulated or round mass
  - Circumscribed margins
  - Calcifications rare
- Atypical or not otherwise specified (NOS) type
  - Borders ill-defined compared to typical medullary carcinoma
Ultrasound Findings
- Typical type
  - Well-defined, hypoechoic mass
  - Large lesions may have anechoic areas
  - Posterior acoustic enhancement not uncommon
- Atypical type
  - Ill-defined margins
  - Posterior acoustic shadowing

Medullary Carcinoma

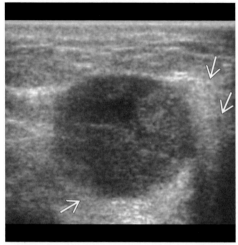

Medullary carcinoma. Ultrasound demonstrates well circumscribed round mass with inhomogeneous internal echoes, an irregular echogenic rim (arrows), and posterior acoustic enhancement.

Differential Diagnosis
Fibroadenoma
Phyllodes
Circumscribed Non-Medullary Breast Cancer

Pathology
General
- General Path Comments
  - Axillary metastases 20-45%
  - Multicentric 8-10 %
  - Typically estrogen and progesterone receptor negative
  - Typically no HER 2/neu reactivity
  - Strict histologic criteria adherence important for management decisions

Gross Pathological, Surgical Features
- Median size 2-3 cm
- Well-defined expansile mass
- Softer than most breast carcinomas
- Pale brown or gray color
- Cut edge reveals nodular architecture
- Hemorrhage and necrosis

Microscopic Features
- Typical type
  - Invasive tumor contains no glandular elements
  - Intense lymphoplasmacytic reaction
  - Syncytial growth pattern with "pushing" borders
  - Poorly-differentiated nuclear grade
  - High mitotic rate
  - Minimal desmoplastic stromal reaction
- Atypical type
  - Fails to meet strict criteria for typical type

Medullary Carcinoma

- o Foci of infiltrating ductal carcinoma not otherwise specified (NOS)
- o Little or no lymphoplasmacytic reaction

Clinical Issues
Presentation
- Most lesions palpable
  - o Soft
  - o Mobile
  - o Usually in upper outer quadrant
  - o May be perceived as benign
- Core biopsy
  - o Sampling may allow only suggestion of diagnosis
- Axillary lymph nodes may be large even in absence of nodal metastases

Treatment
- Standard surgical cancer treatment: Mastectomy
  - o Lumpectomy and radiation therapy
    - Limited reported experience
  - o Axillary or sentinel node dissection
  - o Chemotherapy based on size and nodal status

Prognosis
- Typical form
  - o Survival may be better than infiltrating ductal carcinoma NOS
- Atypical form
  - o Same as other NOS infiltrating carcinomas

Selected References
1. Wong SL et al: Frequency of sentinel lymph node metastases in patients with favorable breast cancer histologic subtypes. Am J Surg 184:492-8, 2002
2. Cheung YL et al: Sonographic and pathological findings in typical and atypical medullary carcinomas of the breast. J Clin Ultrasound 28; 325-31, 2000
3. Cook DL et al: Comparison of DNA content, S-Phase fraction, and medullary and ductal carcinoma of the breast. J Clin Path 104(1):17-22, 1995

Metaplastic Carcinoma

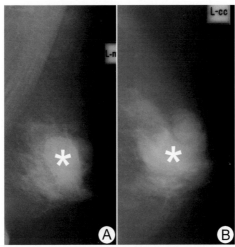

Adenocarcinoma with osteosarcomatous metaplasia. (A) Left MLO and (B) Left CC mammograms show a well-defined, lobulated, uncalcified, dense, rounded mass (*). There was also a large palpable mass clinically. No calcifications were seen on magnification views.

Key Facts
- Synonyms: Adenosquamous carcinoma, squamous carcinoma, carcinosarcoma, mucoepidermoid carcinoma, carcinoma with sarcomatous metaplasia, sarcomatoid carcinoma, adenoacanthoma sarcomatoides
- Definition: Adenocarcinoma mixed with other epithelial or mesenchymal neoplastic elements
- Classification: Squamous, pseudosarcomatous
- Classic imaging appearance
  - Large breast mass, usually well defined; may have ossification
- Other key facts
  - Special uncommon carcinoma variants
  - May be confused with true sarcomas

Imaging Findings
General Features
- Best imaging clue: Uptake of bone scan isotope (e.g., Tc99m-MDP) in breast mass (chondro-osseous and osteosarcomatous types)
- Usually no specific imaging findings
- Shape: Rounded, lobulated or irregular
- Size range: 1 to 20 cm, mean 3-5 cm
- Vector of spread: Lymph nodes, hematogenous
Mammography Findings
- Well-defined, lobulated or irregular nodular mass
- Absent, subtle or (rarely) prominent calcification or ossification
Ultrasound Findings
- Hypoechoic, fairly well-defined mass
- May be hypervascular on color Doppler

Metaplastic Carcinoma

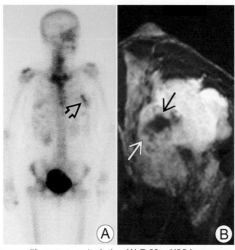

Adenocarcinoma with osseous metaplasia. (A) Tc99m-MDP bone scan shows tumor tracer uptake indicating osteoblastic activity (arrow). (B) Fat-suppressed sagittal post-gadolinium MRI shows large, smoothly-marginated, intensely enhancing mass. Nearby slices show less-enhanced heterogeneous part of tumor (arrows).

MR Findings
- T1 C- – nonspecific mass isointense with breast tissue
- T2WI – nonspecific mass hypointense to breast tissue
- T1 C+ – markedly hyperintense rapid enhancement, typical for malignancy; lobulated mass, no specific features

Imaging Recommendations
- Role of imaging: Localization, image-guided biopsy, staging
- Bone scan useful for staging in chondro-osseous, osteosarcomatous type
- No specific advantage for any other modality

Differential Diagnosis

Malignant Phyllodes Tumor
- Also large rapidly growing mass
- May have sarcomatous elements
- Distinct microscopic growth pattern

Papilloma With Squamous Metaplasia
- Presentation & imaging usually differ
- Primarily pathological differential diagnosis

Breast Metastasis from Remote Malignancy
- Squamous carcinoma or sarcoma

Primary Breast Sarcoma
- Pure sarcomatous stromal tumor without adenocarcinoma
- Arises from mesenchymal elements only
- Spindle cell metaplasia difficult to distinguish from fibrosarcoma, malignant fibrous histiocytoma – cytokeratin positive, squamous nests
- Immunohistochemistry differs

Metaplastic Carcinoma

Pathology
General
- General Path Comments
  - Epithelial and/or myoepithelial cell origins
  - Variable cell composition; named by dominant cell type
  - Suspect if mixed malignant cells in fine needle aspirate or core biopsy
- Etiology-Pathogenesis: Unknown
- Epidemiology
  - Usually women > 50, age range 20-90
  - 16% medullary carcinoma
  - 3.7% ductal carcinoma
  - Pseudosarcomatous metaplasia in 0.2% of adenocarcinomas

Gross Pathologic, Surgical Features
- Solid firm to hard nodular mass +/− cystic degeneration (squamous)

Microscopic Features
- Two major types: Squamous and pseudosarcomatous
- Squamous types
  - Focal squamous large cell nests in adenocarcinoma; purely squamous carcinoma; intermixed in adenosquamous
  - Spindle-cell: Extensive spindle cell component; may appear purely spindle-cell, always cytokeratin positive (rare in fibrosarcoma)
  - Pseudoangiosarcomatous/angiomatoid: Large spaces lined by cytokeratin positive cells (cf. Factor VIII or CD34 in angiosarcoma)
- Pseudosarcomatous
  - Matrix-producing (chondrosarcomatous, chondro-osseous or osteosarcomatous): Poorly-differentiated adenocarcinoma with areas of chondroid differentiation and/or bone formation
  - Very rarely rhabdomyosarcomatous, liposarcomatous, angiosarcomatous forms

Staging and Grading
- Nodal and distant metastases usually absent at diagnosis

Clinical Issues
Presentation
- Females, peak incidence > 55
- Usually large palpable mass

Natural History
- May grow very rapidly or be stable and low grade for years
- 50% hematogenous spread eventually

Treatment
- As for ductal carcinoma; limited chemotherapy and tamoxifen response

Prognosis
- Uncertain for many cases; low grade has good prognosis and survival
- May have higher mortality than ductal carcinoma
  - Especially high-grade spindle cell type

Selected References
1. Kurian KM et al: Sarcomatoid/metaplastic carcinoma of the breast: A clinicopathological study of 12 cases. Histopathology 40:58-64, 2002
2. Park JM et al: Metaplastic carcinoma of the breast: Mammographic and sonographic findings. J Clin Ultrasound 28:179-86, 2000
3. Rayson D et al: Metaplastic breast cancer: Prognosis and response to systemic therapy. Ann Oncol 10:413-9, 1999

Metastases To Breast

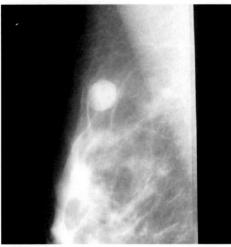

Metastatic melanoma to the breast. Mammogram shows round, smooth, well-circumscribed upper breast mass without associated distortion or calcifications.

Key Facts
- Definition: Involvement of the breast by metastatic disease from other primary malignancies
- Classic imaging appearance: Round, solitary, well-circumscribed peripheral mass in upper outer quadrant
- Isolated metastasis to breast rare
  - Other sites of metastasis usually present
- 3 different types
  - Cross-lymphatic from contralateral breast (most common)
  - Hematogenous
    - Melanoma
    - Lung cancer
    - Soft-tissue sarcomas
    - Ovarian
    - Other (stomach, kidney, cervix, thyroid, colon, uterus)
    - Prostate in males
  - Hematologic malignancy
    - Lymphoma/leukemia

Imaging Findings
General Features
- Best imaging clue: Solitary, well-defined, superficial, discrete mass in upper outer quadrant
Mammography Findings
- Hematogenous
  - Round, well-circumscribed, noncalcified mass
  - Predilection for upper outer quadrant
  - Solitary mass most common (initial presentation)
  - Multiple & bilateral masses (later as disease progresses)
  - Spiculation rare
  - Calcifications rare

Metastases To Breast

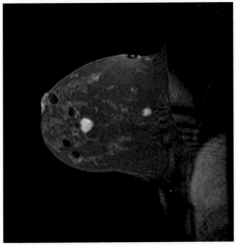

Metastatic melanoma to the breast. T1 C+ MR image shows two fairly well-defined enhancing masses

- ▪ Ovarian/medullary thyroid metastases
- Cross-lymphatics
  - o Skin thickening/peau d'orange/skin nodules
- Hematologic malignancy
  - o Multiple, infiltrative irregular unilateral or bilateral masses
  - o Asymmetric densities
  - o Axillary adenopathy

Ultrasound Findings
- Round/ovoid solid mass with some lobulation
  - o Margins smooth or irregular
- Variable internal echoes
  - o May be almost anechoic
- Posterior acoustic enhancement not common

T1 C+ MR Findings
- Round, well-circumscribed or ill-defined, rim-enhancing mass

Imaging Recommendations
- Biopsy if management will be altered
  - o To distinguish primary breast from metastasis

Differential Diagnosis
Primary Breast Carcinoma
- Medullary, mucinous or papillary (well circumscribed)

Cyst
- Ultrasound will usually make diagnosis

Fibroadenoma
- Ultrasound may be sufficient
- Biopsy

Pathology
General
- General Path Comments

- o In situ, ductal, lobular absent in metastatic non-breast primary lesion
- Etiology-Pathogenesis
  - o Contralateral breast carcinoma spreads via cross-lymphatics
  - o Extramammary tumor via hematogenous spread
  - o Hematologic malignancy
- Epidemiology
  - o Rare: 0.5–3% of all breast malignancies

Microscopic Features
- Periductal or perilobular malignant cells
- No in situ carcinoma

Staging or Grading Criteria
- Stage IV

Clinical Issues
Presentation
- Cross-lymphatic spread
  - o Skin thickening/peau d'orange/skin nodules
- Hematologic spread
  - o Firm painless mobile mass
- Hematologic malignancy
  - o Axillary adenopathy
- Antecedent history of primary malignancy suggests diagnosis
- Rapid growth suggests diagnosis

Treatment
- Systemic treatment appropriate to primary lesion
- Mastectomy appropriate for local control of bulky/symptomatic disease
- Lymph node dissection for local control

Prognosis
- Extremely poor generally
- Depends on characteristics of specific malignancy

Selected References
1.   Toombs BD et al: Metastatic disease to the breast: Clinical, pathologic, and radiographic features. AJR 129:673-6, 1997
2.   Derchi LE e al: Metastatic tumors in the breast: Sonographic findings. J Ultrasound Med 4:69-74, 1985
3.   McCrea ES et al: Metastases to the breast. AJR 141:685-90, 1983

Mucinous Carcinoma

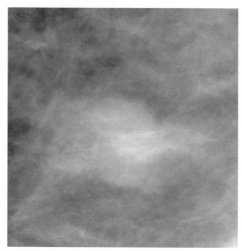

Mucinous carcinoma. 43-year-old woman with palpable 3 o'clock right breast lump. Mammogram: Spot magnified MLO view demonstrates an ill-defined, partially-circumscribed mass.

Key Facts
- Synonyms: Colloid carcinoma, gelatinous carcinoma
- Definition: Well-differentiated, invasive adenocarcinoma
  - Tumor cells in lakes of mucin
- Classic imaging appearance
  - Round, fairly well-circumscribed mass
- Other key facts
  - More common in postmenopausal women
  - Slow growing
  - More favorable prognosis than other infiltrating carcinomas not otherwise specified (NOS)
  - Pure
    - > 75% mucinous cells
  - Mixed
    - Mucinous and invasive NOS elements

Imaging Findings
Mammography Findings
- Pure type
  - Circumscribed lobular mass
  - Calcifications rare
- Mixed type
  - Irregular mass
  - Ill-defined margins

Ultrasound Findings
- Variable mass characteristics
  - Well-circumscribed ill-defined
- Posterior acoustic features

Mucinous Carcinoma

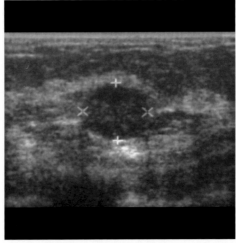

Mucinous carcinoma. Ultrasound. Well-circumscribed, round, hypoechoic mass with posterior acoustic enhancement. Careful evaluation of the margins demonstrated no thin, echogenic, surrounding rim.

- o Enhancement
- o Shadowing

<u>MR Findings</u>
- Well-defined, round, enhancing mass
- Lobulated border
- Homogeneous enhancement
- May have internal enhancing septations

Differential Diagnosis
<u>Fibroadenoma</u>
<u>Papilloma</u>
<u>Mucin-Containing Cyst</u>

Pathology
<u>General</u>
- General Path Comments
  - o < 5% of breast cancers
  - o Pure type usually smaller than mixed type
  - o Axillary metastases
    - Pure form = 10%
    - Mixed form = 40%
  - o Estrogen/progesterone receptor in pure form
    - ER = 92%
    - PR = 68%

<u>Gross Pathologic, Surgical Features</u>
- 1-20 cm
- Circumscribed expansile mass
- Moist, glistening, cut surface
- Soft and gelatinous
  - o May be firm to hard

Mucinous Carcinoma

Microscopic Features
- Aggregates of tumor cells surrounded by mucin
  - Cellular arrangement
    - Slender strands
    - Papillary clusters
    - Compartmentalized by fibrovascular bands
- Gland formation uncommon
- May be associated with low-grade ductal carcinoma in situ

Clinical Issues
Presentation
- Soft on palpation
  - May be perceived as benign
- Often image detected
- Core biopsy more reliable than fine needle aspiration
Treatment
- Standard surgical cancer treatment
  - Lumpectomy and radiation therapy
  - Mastectomy
  - Axillary or sentinel node dissection
  - Chemotherapy based on size and nodal status
Prognosis
- Pure form
  - Excellent
- Mixed form
  - Same as other NOS infiltrating carcinomas

Selected References
1. Kawashima M: MR imaging of mucinous carcinoma of the breast. AJR 179:179-83, 2002
2. Paramo JC et al: Pure mucinous carcinoma of the breast; is axillary staging necessary? Ann Surg Oncol 9:161-4, 2002
3. Renshaw AA: Can mucinous lesions of the breast be reliably diagnosed by core needle biopsy? AMJ Clin Pathol 118:82-4, 2002

Non-Hodgkin's Lymphoma

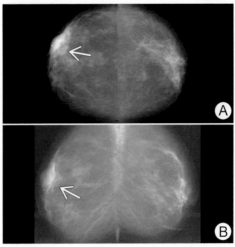

Non-Hodgkin's B-cell lymphoma. 50-year-old women with palpable right retroareolar mass. Note partially obscured mass on mammogram (arrow) (A) Bilateral CC view. (B) Bilateral MLO views.

Key Facts
- Definition
  - Primary
    - Breast documented as principal organ involved and primary site
    - No evidence of antecedent extramammary lymphoma
  - Secondary
    - Involvement of breast tissue associated with systemic or nodal disease at other sites
- Classic imaging appearance
  - Uncalcified, well-circumscribed mass
- Accounts for less than 0.5% of all breast cancers
- Average age at diagnosis 55 years
- Bilaterality 10-15%
- Right-sided predominance 60:40
- Two principle patterns of primary disease
  - Diffuse large cell type (most common)
    - B-cell origin
    - Unilateral
    - Broad age range
    - Variable course
  - Burkitt's type
    - Younger women
    - Pregnant or lactating
    - Bilateral
    - Rapidly fatal course
    - Ovarian metastases
    - May progress to lymphoblastic leukemia

Non-Hodgkin's Lymphoma

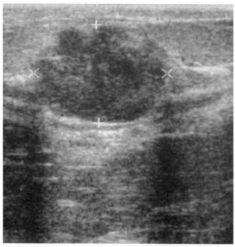

Non-Hodgkin's lymphoma. Same case as previous page. Ultrasound of biopsy – proven non-Hodgkin's lymphoma. Lobulated, oval hypoechoic mass with prominent posterior acoustic enhancement.

Imaging Findings
Mammography Findings
- Solitary noncalcified mass
  - Well-circumscribed, lobulated or ill-defined margins
  - No spiculation
- Multiple noncalcified masses
  - More common in secondary involvement
  - 10% in primary involvement
- Diffuse increased opacity with skin thickening

Ultrasound Findings
- Hypoechoic well-defined mass
  - Low amplitude echoes
  - May be almost anechoic in some cases
    - Meticulous US technique to avoid misdiagnosing as simple cyst
- Enhancement characteristics variable

Imaging Recommendations
- Mammography and ultrasound in all patients
- Ga-67 scintigraphy
  - Intense accumulation in both primary and secondary lymphoma
  - Helpful in confirmation of diagnosis
  - Demonstrates extent of systemic involvement
  - Valuable in assessing therapeutic response in follow-up patients

Differential Diagnosis
Pseudolymphoma
- Presents as solid, firm mass with fat necrosis
- Lymphoid infiltrate has no atypical cells
  - Often displays germinal centers
- May present as an overwhelming response to injury

Non-Hodgkin's Lymphoma

Pathology
General
- May be mistaken for carcinoma, with needle biopsies (fine needle aspiration or core) and on frozen section
- Size range 1-12 cm; average 3cm
- Estrogen and progesterone positivity have been reported
- Etiology-Pathogenesis
  o Thought to arise from periductal or perilobular lymphoid tissue

Gross Pathologic, Surgical Features
- Circumscribed fleshy tumor
- Cut surface gray-white to pink
- Softening and brown discoloration indicative of necrosis

Microscopic Features
- Lymphomatous infiltrate extends beyond grossly evident mass
- Uniform population of tumor cells
- Ducts and lobules may be partially or completely obliterated in central portion of tumor

Clinical Issues
Presentation
- Usually presents with palpable mass
  o Often painful
  o Rapid growth
- Skin fixation with cutaneous inflammatory changes in some cases
  o Must differentiate from locally advanced breast cancer
- Axillary involvement 30-50%
  o Adenopathy softer than that associated with carcinoma
- Night sweats, fever, weight loss 10%

Treatment
- Standard surgical cancer treatment
  o Lumpectomy/radiation therapy or mastectomy
  o Axillary lymph node dissection
- Adjuvant chemotherapy
  o Intermediate to high grade
    ▪ CHOP-Cytoxan, Adriamycin, vincristine, prednisone
- Relapse of primary breast lymphoma
  o High dose chemotherapy
  o Stem cell rescue

Prognosis
- Overall 5-year survival 46-85%

Selected References
1. Wong WW et al: Primary Non-Hodgkin's lymphoma of the breast: The Mayo Clinic experience. Jour Surg Onc 80(1):19-25, 2002
2. Zach JR: Primary breast lymphoma originating in a benign intramammary lymph node. AJR 177:177-8, 2001
3. Liberman L et al: Non-Hodgkin's lymphoma of the breast: Imaging characteristics and correlation with histopathologic findings. Radiology 194:157-60, 1994

Paget's Disease of the Nipple

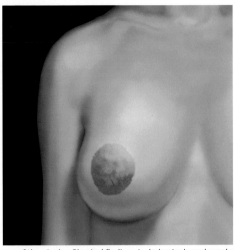

Paget's disease of the nipple. Physical findings include nipple and areolar thickening, reddening and scaling, pruritis, and ulceration.

Key Facts
- Definition: An uncommon variant of ductal carcinoma in situ (DCIS)
  - Malignant cells extend to nipple surface through lactiferous ducts
  - Characteristic skin changes clue to diagnosis
- Classic imaging appearance
  - Nipple and areolar thickening
- Other key facts
  - 1-5% of all breast cancers
  - 50% have underlying palpable mass
  - Associated carcinoma found in breast or nipple in 95%
  - Median age 56-62 years
  - Less than 5% of male breast cancers
    - Associated with Klinefelter's syndrome

Imaging Findings
Mammography Findings
- Nipple and areola thickening
- Nipple retraction
- Subareolar mass or calcifications
- Mass or calcifications away from nipple
- May severely underestimate extent of disease
- May be normal in 50%
Ultrasound Findings
- Paget's disease per se not identified on ultrasound
- Underlying carcinoma may appear as any other malignant lesion
Imaging Recommendations
- Mammography in all patients
- Ultrasound selected patients
  - Palpable mass

Paget's Disease of the Nipple

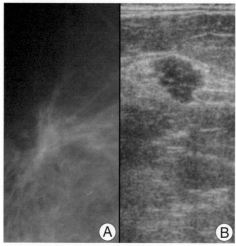

Paget's disease of the nipple. Ultrasound of RUOQ architectural distortion identified on mammography (A) shows ill-defined hypoechoic mass with no acoustic enhancement or shadowing (B). Biopsy infiltrating ductal carcinoma.

- o Abnormality on mammogram
- o Dense breast tissue on mammogram (controversial)

Differential Diagnosis

Clinical
- Eczema
- Nipple adenoma
  - o Erosion, ulceration and nipple enlargement
- Protruding intraductal papilloma
  - o Weeping, red lesion

Pathological
- Malignant melanoma
- Florid ductal papillomatosis
- Squamous or basal cell carcinoma
- Nipple adenoma

Pathology

General
- General Path Comments
  - o Most DCIS associated = high grade, comedo, or solid type
    - ▪ May be associated with invasion or exist alone
  - o Axillary lymph node involvement
    - ▪ With palpable mass 20-69%
    - ▪ Without palpable mass 8-29%
  - o Rare cases reported without underlying DCIS or invasive carcinoma
    - ▪ DCIS arises from ductal epithelium at squamocolumnar duct junction

Gross Pathologic, Surgical Features
- Duplicate those seen clinically
- Occasionally enlarged lactiferous ducts

Paget's Disease of the Nipple

- Underlying palpable tumors have no specific features

Microscopic Features
- Paget's cells (adenocarcinoma) in keratinizing epithelium of nipple epidermis
- Abundant pale or clear cytoplasm
- Large nuclei with prominent nucleoli
- Melanin pigment may be present

Clinical Issues
Presentation
- Initial
  - Reddening and/or scaling of nipple and areola
  - Pruritus
- Progression
  - Moist, scaling, eczematous changes
  - Ulceration, crusting and erosion of nipple
  - Serous or bloody nipple discharge
- Mimics benign dermatological conditions
  - Inflammatory component can be improved with topical treatment
  - May result in delay in diagnosis
- Diagnosis
  - Wedge biopsy
  - Shave and punch biopsy less reliable

Treatment
- Standard
  - Mastectomy with axillary node biopsy/dissection
    - Extensive DCIS
    - Close margins in a nipple-areolar biopsy specimen
- Selected cases
  - Breast conservation and radiation therapy
    - Limited extent of underlying DCIS
    - No associated palpable mass
- Axillary dissection not indicated for limited DCIS
- Chemotherapy
  - Invasive
    - Same treatment criteria as for other infiltrating ductal carcinomas
  - DCIS
    - Typically not used

Prognosis
- Excellent when DCIS only
- Determined by stage of invasive cancer

Selected References
1. Bijker N: Breast conserving therapy for Paget's disease of the nipple: A prospective European organization for research and treatment of cancer study of 61 Patients. Cancer 91(3):472-7, 2001
2. Burke ET: Paget's disease of the breast: A pictorial essay. Radiographics 18(6):1459-64, 1998
3. Ikeda DM: Paget's disease of the nipple: Radiologic-pathologic correlation. Radiology 189:89-94, 1993

Sarcomas

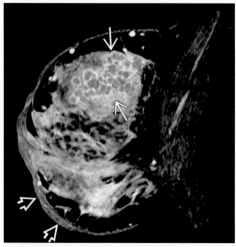

Sarcoma. T1 C+ MRI shows an extensive left breast rapidly enhancing 11 cm angiosarcoma with chest wall invasion (not shown) and extensive skin thickening (open arrows). Much of the mass demonstrated homogeneous enhancement while portions showed multiple areas of rim enhancement (arrows).

Key Facts
- Definition: Malignant stromal breast neoplasms
- Classic imaging appearance
  - Fairly well-defined mammographic or sonographic mass
- Other key facts
  - < 1% of all malignant breast lesions
  - May have well-circumscribed margins
  - Some types associated with past history of radiation therapy
  - Imaging of limited benefit to differentiate from other lesions

Imaging Findings
Mammography Findings
- Angiosarcoma
  - Lobulated or ill-defined mass
  - Average size = 5 cm
- Osteogenic sarcoma
  - Well-defined or irregular mass
  - May have calcifications
  - Average size = 10 cm
- Malignant fibrous histiocytoma
  - Fairly well circumscribed
  - Lobulated
  - Average size = 7 cm
- Others reported
  - Liposarcoma
  - Fibrosarcoma
  - Leiomyosarcoma
  - Hemangiopericytoma
  - Rhabdomyosarcoma
  - Malignant peripheral nerve sheath tumors

Sarcomas

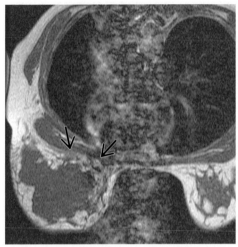

Sarcoma. T1 axial image of the same case as previous image shows the left breast to be larger than the right and evidence of tumor extension into the chest wall (arrows). No axillary or internal mammary adenopathy was seen.

<u>Ultrasound Findings</u>
- Focal masses
- Variable internal echogenicity
- Nonspecific findings

<u>MR Findings</u>
- Post T1 C+
  - Nonspecific, focal, enhancing mass
  - Some well-rounded with well-defined margins
  - May have heterogeneous internal enhancement

Differential Diagnosis

<u>Benign Lesions</u>
- Imaging may simulate benign lesions
  - Fibroadenomas
  - Phyllodes

<u>Invasive Ductal Carcinoma</u>
- Imaging characteristics may be identical

<u>Metaplastic Carcinoma</u>
- Mammary carcinomas with metaplasia
- Microscopic changes diverge from glandular differentiation
  - Squamous metaplasia
  - Sarcomatoid metaplasia
- Most difficult distinction
  - Fibrosarcoma vs. metaplastic spindle-cell squamous carcinoma

Pathology

<u>General</u>
- Very rare
  - Angiosarcoma most common
- Etiology-Pathogenesis

Sarcomas

- Relationship to radiation exposure
  - Angiosarcoma
  - Malignant fibrous histiocytoma
  - Fibrosarcoma

Gross Pathologic, Surgical Features
- Large masses

Microscopic Features
- Angiosarcoma
  - Type 1
    - Anastomosing vascular channels
  - Type 2
    - Cellular proliferations projecting into vascular channels
  - Type 3
    - Endothelial tufting, mitoses, necrosis
- Osteogenic sarcoma
  - Associations with other histologies
    - Chondrosarcoma
    - High-grade spindle-cell sarcoma
  - Multinucleated osteoclastic giant cells
- Malignant fibrous histiocytoma
  - Spindle cells arranged in a pinwheel pattern

Clinical Issues
Presentation
- Palpable mass
- Angiosarcoma associated with bluish skin discoloration

Treatment
- Mastectomy most common
- Axillary dissection typically not performed
  - Axillary metastases rare

Prognosis
- Variable
- Based on tissue type and grade
  - Fairly good to poor range

Selected References
1. Mazaki R et al: Liposarcoma of the breast; a case report and review of the literature. Int Surg 87:164-70, 2002
2. Rosen PP: Breast pathology: Diagnosis by needle core biopsy. Lippincott Williams & Wikins, Philadelphia PA. Chapter 23, 234-40, 1999
3. Borman H et al: Fibrosarcoma following radiotherapy for breast carcinoma: A case report and review of the literature. Ann Plast Surg 41:201-4, 1998

Tubular Carcinoma

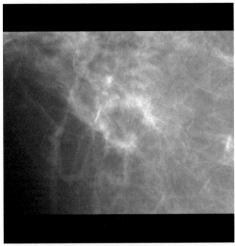

Tubular carcinoma. 52-year-old asymptomatic woman. Screening mammogram detects questionable lesion in the right upper inner quadrant. Rolled CC view demonstrates 8 mm spiculated mass with associated architectural distortion.

Key Facts
- Synonym: Well differentiated carcinoma
- Definition: Most well differentiated form of infiltrating ductal carcinoma
- Classic imaging appearance
  - Small spiculated mass on mammogram
- Indistinguishable from infiltrating ductal carcinoma (IDC)
  - Not otherwise specified (NOS)
- < 5% of breast cancers
- More favorable prognosis than IDC NOS
- Median age 48
  - Slightly younger than IDC NOS

Imaging Findings
Mammography Findings
- Small spiculated mass
- Round or oval mass
- Architectural distortion
- Asymmetric density
- Microcalcifications

Ultrasound Findings
- Ill-defined hypoechoic mass
- Posterior acoustic shadowing
- Hyperechoic foci representing calcifications may be seen

MR Findings
- Enhancement characteristics typical for invasive ductal carcinoma
  - Irregular spiculated mass
  - Strong rapid contrast enhancement
  - Rim enhancement
  - Inhomogeneous enhancement

Tubular Carcinoma

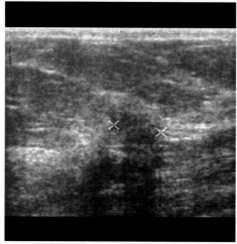

Tubular carcinoma. Ultrasound reveals corresponding irregular hypoechoic mass with posterior acoustic shadowing.

- May show benign-type enhancement pattern

Differential Diagnosis
Radial Scar
- Spiculated mass on mammography
  - May contain central lucent area
  - Long spicules
- Architectural distortion
- Histology
  - Distorted ducts
  - Surrounding fibrosis and elastosis
  - Two cell-layer ducts
- Core biopsy or frozen section histology
  - May not fully differentiate from tubular carcinoma
Sclerosing Adenosis
- Ill-defined mass on mammography
- Punctate calcifications may be associated
- No typical sonographic appearance
- Histology
  - Glands with double cell layers
  - Epithelial and myoepithelial cells
  - Lobular pattern

Pathology
General
- General Path Comments
  - Lower incidence of axillary lymph node metastasis
  - Multicentric up to 28%
  - Bilateral 12-40%
  - 1% of male breast cancers

Tubular Carcinoma

Gross Pathologic, Surgical Features
- 1-2 cm
- Tan-to-gray cut surface
- Ill-defined or spiculated margins
- Firm

Microscopic Features
- Well-formed tubular elements
- Single cell lining
  - No myoepithelial cells
- Uniform nuclei
- Low mitotic rate
- Abundant cytoplasm
  - Luminal projections ("snouts")
- Associated with noncomedo ductal carcinoma in situ
  - 2/3 cases

Clinical Issues

Presentation
- Most image detected
- May be palpable

Natural History
- Slow growing

Treatment
- Lumpectomy
- Axillary or sentinel node dissection
- Radiation therapy and chemotherapy
  - Less frequent than other invasive cancers

Prognosis
- 95% five-year survival

Selected References
1.   Sheppard DG: Tubular carcinoma of the breast: Mammographic and sonographic features. AJR 174:253-7, 2000
2.   Mitnik JS: Tubular carcinoma of the breast: Sensitivity of diagnostic techniques and correlation with histopathology. AJR 172:319-23, 1999
3.   Bassett LW et al: Diagnosis of diseases of the breast. Philadelphia: WB Saunders Co. Chapter 27, 489-91, 1997

Tubulolobular Carcinoma

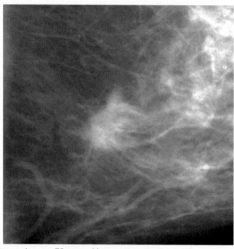

Tubulolobular carcinoma. 70-year-old asymptomatic woman. Screening mammogram: Standard CC view of left breast. Spiculated mass at medial fat-mammary interface.

Key Facts
- Definition: A rare type of infiltrating breast cancer
  - Histological features of both tubular and lobular carcinoma
- Classic imaging appearance
  - Characteristics of both tubular and infiltrating lobular carcinoma
- Other key facts
  - Less favorable prognosis than tubular carcinoma
  - Younger age group than other breast cancers
    - Average age 42

Imaging Findings
Mammography Findings
- Variable
  - Round circumscribed mass, spiculated mass
Ultrasound Findings
- Well-circumscribed to ill-defined hypoechoic mass
- Posterior acoustic shadowing

Differential Diagnosis
Tubular Carcinoma
Lobular Carcinoma
Radial Scar

Pathology
General
- Multifocal = 29%
- Axillary lymph node metastasis = 43%
- Associated lobular carcinoma in situ (LCIS) = 35%
- Mean size 1.3 cm
- Estrogen receptor positive

Tubulolobular Carcinoma

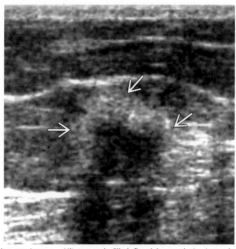

Tubulolobular carcinoma. Ultrasound: Ill-defined hypoechoic, irregular, mass not oriented parallel to the skin with a thick echogenic rim (arrows) and posterior acoustic shadowing.

- Progesterone receptor positive

Gross Pathologic, Surgical Features
- Ill-defined, firm, gray mass
- Stellate appearance of cut surface
  o Similar to radial scar

Microscopic Features
- Admixture of tubular glands and cords of small uniform cells in linear pattern
- Low mitotic activity; low nuclear grade
- Intracytoplasmic vacuoles
- Apocrine cells present

Clinical Issues

Presentation
- Often detected on screening mammogram
- Core biopsy

Treatment
- Standard surgical cancer treatment
- Lumpectomy and radiation therapy
- Mastectomy
- Axillary or sentinel node dissection
- Chemotherapy based on size and nodal status

Prognosis
- Good
  o Intermediate between pure tubular and invasive lobular carcinoma

Selected References
1.   Rosen P: Tubular carcinoma. Rosen's breast pathology, 2nd edition. 370-5, 2001
2.   Green I: A Comparative study of pure tubular and tubulolobular carcinoma of the breast. Am J Surg Path. 21(6):653-7, 1997
3.   Boppana S: Cytologic Characteristics of tubulolobular carcinoma of the breast. Acta Cytologica. 40(3):465-71, 1996

PocketRadiologist®
Breast
Top 100 Diagnoses

THE MALE BREAST

Gynecomastia

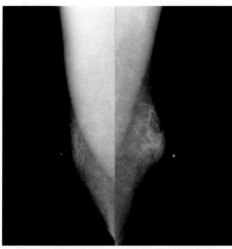

Gynecomastia. 58-year-old man with asymmetric breast enlargement, left larger than right. Bilateral MLO mammogram shows left retroareolar tissue without worrisome mass. Patient was taking antihypertensive medication, likely the cause of this unilateral gynecomastia. Note the large pectoralis muscles.

Key Facts
- Definition: Nonneoplastic enlargement of male breast
- Classic imaging appearance: Flame-shaped retroareolar mass
- Most common clinical & pathological abnormality of male breast

Imaging Findings
General Features
- Best imaging clue: Flame-shaped subareolar density extending into upper outer quadrant

Mammography Findings
- Two patterns
  - Nodular, flame-shaped
    - Triangular/conical density in subareolar region
    - Associated with florid histological pattern
  - Dendritic
    - Prominent radial extensions into breast
    - Associated with fibrous histological pattern
- Bilateral > unilateral
- Asymmetric > symmetric
- No associated calcifications

Ultrasound Findings
- Typically hypoechoic regions reflecting mammographic configuration
- Hypoechoic findings likened to shape of a hand with wrist at level of the nipple and "fingers" seen as extensions into relatively hyperechoic surrounding tissue

Imaging Recommendations
- Two-view bilateral mammography

Gynecomastia

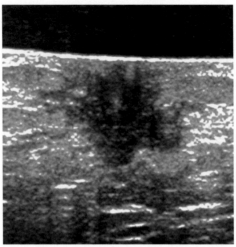

Gynecomastia subareolar ultrasound. Fibroglandular tissue is hypoechoic. Some have likened this appearance to the shape of a hand with the "wrist" at the nipple level and the "palm and fingers" extending as hypoechoic structures into the tissue deep to the nipple-areolar complex.

Differential Diagnosis

Male Breast Cancer
- Mass usually present

Pseudogynecomastia
- Fatty enlargement
- No glandular tissue

Diabetic Mastopathy
- Palpable mass
- Within fibroglandular tissue (gynecomastia)

Lipoma
- Radiolucency on mammography with thin capsule
- May have negative mammogram

Pathology

General
- General Path Comments
  - Abnormal increase in stromal & ductal components
  - Florid type (reversible) within 1 year of onset
    - Increased ducts with epithelial hyperplasia
    - Increased vascularity of surrounding stroma
    - Edema
  - Fibrous type (irreversible) usually after 6 months or longer
    - Increased ducts with little epithelial proliferation
    - Fibrotic & hyalinized stroma
    - Reduced vascularity
- Etiology-Pathogenesis
  - Associated with increased estrogen and decreased testosterone
- Epidemiology
  - 85% of breast masses in males

Gynecomastia

- o Tri-modal distribution (newborns, adolescents & older men)
- o Causes (numerous)
  - Hormonal (puberty: ↑ estradiol; older men: ↓ testosterone)
  - Drug-induced (estrogen treatment for prostate cancer, digitalis, cimetidine, spironolactone, thiazide, reserpine, marijuana, isoniazid, ergotamine, tricyclic antidepressants)
  - Systemic disorders (chronic renal failure, liver cirrhosis, chronic pulmonary disease, adrenal & thyroid disease, diabetes, Klinefelter's syndrome, testicular feminization, hypogonadism, hyperthyroidism, refeeding after starvation)
  - Tumors (pulmonary carcinoma, hepatoma, adrenal carcinoma, pituitary adenoma, testicular germ cell tumors)
  - Idiopathic

Gross Pathologic, Surgical Features
- Soft rubbery or firm gray/white tissue forms mass or area of induration
- Fat rarely dispersed in fibrous tissue

Microscopic Features
- Increased number of ducts
- Proliferation of duct epithelium
- Periductal edema
- Fibroblastic stroma
- Adipose tissue

Clinical Issues

Presentation
- Breast enlargement
- May have painful palpable subareolar mass
  - o Usually 2–6 cm
- Rare nipple retraction or discharge

Treatment
- Expectant
- Surgical excision

Prognosis
- Regression described in treated hyperthyroidism & liver cirrhosis
- Usually breast enlargement persists
- May become irreversible if present 6 months or longer
- No increased risk of male breast cancer

Selected References
1. Chantra PK et al: Mammography of the male breast. AJR 164(4):853-8, 1995
2. Dershaw DD: Male mammography. AJR 146(1):127-31, 1986
3. Jackson VP et al: Male breast carcinoma and gynecomastia: Comparison of mammography with sonography. Radiology 149(2):533-6, 1983

Male Breast Cancer

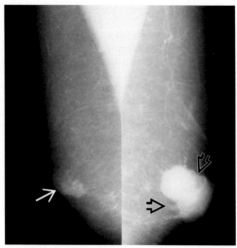

Bilateral MLO views of a 75-year-old man with a history of bilateral gynecomastia (arrow shows gynecomastia of right breast) now with a new palpable left breast mass. Mammogram demonstrates lobulated retroareolar mass in the left breast (open arrows). Pathology yielded infiltrating ductal carcinoma.

Key Facts
- Definition: Carcinoma in male breast
- Classic imaging appearance: Subareolar lobulated uncalcified mass
- < 1% breast cancer

Imaging Findings
<u>Mammography Findings</u>
- Mass 80–90%
  - More likely lobulated, well-defined than seen in women
    - Can be spiculated or irregular
  - Usually subareolar
    - Can be eccentric
    - Eccentric location very suspicious for malignancy
- Calcifications up to 30%
  - Less common than in women
  - May be larger
  - Fewer in number
  - More scattered
  - Pleomorphic morphology less common than in women
- Axillary adenopathy may be present
- Florid gynecomastia may mask carcinoma
<u>Ultrasound Findings</u>
- Hypoechoic, irregular, poorly-defined mass with or without shadowing
<u>Imaging Recommendations</u>
- Two-view mammography
- Sonography for any focal mammographic or worrisome palpable findings

Differential Diagnosis
<u>Gynecomastia</u>
- Fan- or flame-shaped density

Male Breast Cancer

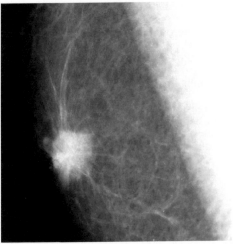

Mammogram. Cone MLO view of a 65-year-old man with palpable fullness in the retroareolar region of the left breast demonstrates a spiculated mass. Pathology = infiltrating ductal carcinoma.

- Extends from subareolar region to upper outer quadrant

<u>Fat Necrosis</u>
- ± spiculated mass
- ± eggshell calcifications

<u>Pseudogynecomastia</u>
- Fatty enlargement of the breast

<u>Granular Cell Tumor</u>
- Spiculated mass

Pathology
<u>General</u>
- General Path Comments
  - 85% = infiltrating ductal carcinoma
  - Associated ductal carcinoma in situ (DCIS) 35–50%
  - Papillary carcinomas more common in men 3–5%
    - Majority intracystic & noninvasive
  - Pure DCIS 10%
  - Infiltrating lobular carcinoma rare
- Genetics
  - Positive family history increases risk to 1.4X normal
  - 30% male breast cancer cases have positive family history
  - Relatives of men with breast cancer have increased risk
    - Equivalent to increase risk with female breast cancer
  - High frequency of BRCA 2 gene (not BRCA 1)
  - Family history of prostate cancer increases risk to 4X normal
- Embryology-Anatomy
  - Male breast does not contain terminal ductal lobular unit (TDLU)
    - Unless stimulated with estrogen
  - Normal male breast contains subareolar ducts with epithelium

Male Breast Cancer

- - Ductal carcinoma can develop
  - o Lobule formation rare (except Klinefelter's/estrogen therapy)
    - Lesions of lobule (fibroadenomas) thus rare
  - o Cyst formation rare
    - May be caused by ductal dilation
- Etiology-Pathogenesis
  - o Ducts give rise to infiltrating ductal carcinoma
- Epidemiology
  - o 0.5–1% of all breast cancer
  - o Higher incidence in men with
    - Prior radiation to the breast
    - Testicular disease (undescended testes, orchidectomy, orchitis, testicular injury)
    - Estrogen use (prostate carcinoma therapy, transsexuals)
    - Systemic (obesity, diabetes, cirrhosis)
  - o Klinefelter's Syndrome
    - Increased risk for developing breast cancer
    - May be associated with gynecomastia (complicating the diagnosis)

Gross Pathologic, Surgical Features
- Identical to female breast

Microscopic Features
- Estrogen receptor positive 85%

Staging or Grading Criteria
- Equivalent to female breast cancer stage for stage

Clinical Issues

Presentation
- Average age at diagnosis 60 yr
- Firm, painless, palpable mass 80–90%
- Nipple changes
  - o Retraction
  - o Ulceration
  - o Discharge
- Paget's disease 2%
- Skin changes may be present
- Axillary adenopathy

Treatment
- Mastectomy & lymph node biopsy/dissection
- Hormonal treatment for metastatic carcinoma

Prognosis
- Equivalent to female breast cancer stage for stage

Selected References
1. Hittmair AP et al: Ductal carcinoma in situ (DCIS) in the male breast: A morphologic study of 84 cases of pure DCIS and 30 cases of DCIS associated with invasive carcinoma - a preliminary report. Cancer 15; 83(10):2139-49, 1998
2. Dershaw DD et al: Mammographic findings in men with breast cancer. AJR 160(2):267-70, 1993
3. Hultborn R et al: Male breast carcinoma. A study of the total material reported to the Swedish Cancer Registry 1958-1967 with respect to clinical and histopathologic parameters. Acta Oncol 26(4):241-56, 1987

PocketRadiologist®
Breast
Top 100 Diagnoses

POST-OP BENIGN

Cosmetic Oil Injections

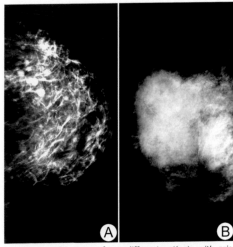

Cosmetic oil injections. CC views of two different patients with prior silicone oil injections. (A) Extensive curvilinear oil deposits along Cooper's ligaments and numerous dense oil droplets in left breast. (B) Extremely dense, calcific granulomas and large, irregular masses in right breast.

Key Facts
- Synonyms: Paraffinoma, silicone mastitis, diffuse silicone granulomas
- Definition: Injection of liquid oil or wax into breast parenchyma for cosmetic augmentation, with foreign body granulomatous reaction
- Classic imaging appearance
  - Silicone granulomas: Extensive, dense, nodular calcifications with variable-sized, radiodense, silicone oil droplets
  - Paraffinoma: Nodular mass(es) with marked fibrotic distortion
- Other key facts
  - Impairs breast evaluation by mammography and ultrasound
  - Paraffin from early 20th century, liquid silicone since 1960s
    - Widespread practice once, now illegal in USA
    - Still used in some parts of Asia

Imaging Findings
General Features With Silicone Injections
- Best imaging clue: Diffuse, very dense, nodular calcifications with linear ductal hyperdensities and sharply-defined hyperdense, round, droplets
- Shape & location: Widespread, throughout entire breast
  - Dependent on injection volume and locations
Mammography Findings
- Innumerable, densely calcified nodules
- Branching, intraductal, hyperdense oil and large oil droplets
Ultrasound Findings
- Irregular hypoechoic areas
- Focal areas with marked shadowing
MR Findings
- T1 C-: Intermediate signal, rounded droplets
- T2WI: Hypointense, mixed intensity areas, or hyperintense oil droplets

Cosmetic Oil Injections

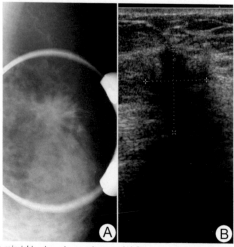

Paraffinoma mimicking invasive carcinoma. (A) Spot compression mammogram shows focal left breast mass with spiculated margins and marked distortion. (B) Ultrasound shows suspicious, hypoechoic, irregular mass with dense shadowing. Paraffinoma diagnosed at core biopsy.

- T1 C+
  - Granulomas show variable enhancement
  - May mimic malignancy
  - Oil droplets nonenhancing

General Features With Paraffin Injections
- Best imaging clue: Focal mass with spiculated margins
- Location: Anywhere in breast
- Size range: 1 to 5 cm

Mammography Findings
- Soft-tissue mass with distortion, no microcalcifications
- May have large, adjacent, circular or flocculent calcifications

Ultrasound Findings
- Hypoechoic, irregular nodule

MR Findings
- T1 C-: Intermediate intensity, irregular mass
- T2WI: Hypointense, irregular mass
- T1 C+: No significant enhancement

Imaging Recommendations (All Oil Injections)
- Mammography and ultrasound may not be useful
- T1 C+ MRI can be useful for diagnosis of breast cancer
- May require MR-guided biopsy procedure

Differential Diagnosis
Invasive Carcinoma (For Paraffinoma)
- May be indistinguishable on conventional imaging
- Often has associated microcalcifications
- Almost always strongly enhancing on MRI

Cosmetic Oil Injections

Pathology

<u>General</u>
- General Path Comments
  - Intense foreign body inflammatory and granulomatous reaction
- Etiology-Pathogenesis
  - Cosmetic injections, usually performed in beauty parlors in Asia
- Epidemiology
  - Almost exclusively Asian patients
  - Paraffinomas reported in male transsexuals

<u>Gross Pathologic, Surgical Features</u>
- Silicone injections
  - Large area of firm, irregular thickening, gritty on bisection
  - Numerous cystic spaces

<u>Microscopic Features</u>
- Diffuse granulomatous reaction with variable fibrosis
- Silicone: Vacuolated spaces containing refractile particles

Clinical Issues

<u>Presentation</u>
- "Lumpy" or hard breast area or mass(es)
- Silicone mastitis may have draining sinuses, ulceration, deformity
- May be discovered at screening mammography
- Patient may deny any past procedure

<u>Natural History</u>
- Paraffinoma: Rarely ulcerates skin
- Silicone oil migrates: Lymph nodes, chest wall, abdomen, groin

<u>Treatment</u>
- Surgical excision or mastectomy if ulcerated or destructive mastitis
- Counseling with expectant management

<u>Prognosis</u>
- Silicone may cause chronic, recurrent, destructive mastitis
- No proven link with autoimmune diseases
- No proven increase in breast cancer incidence

Selected References
1. Wang J et al: Magnetic resonance imaging characteristics of paraffinomas and siliconomas after mammoplasty. J Formos Med Assoc 101:117-23, 2002
2. Caskey CI et al: Imaging spectrum of extracapsular silicone: Correlation of US, MR imaging, mammographic, and histopathologic findings. Radiographics 19 Spec No:S39-51, 1999
3. Yang WT et al: Paraffinomas of the breast: Mammographic, ultrasonographic and radiographic appearances with clinical and histopathological correlation. Clin Radiol 51:130-3, 1996

Implant Saline

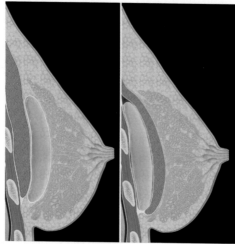

Implant saline. Diagram shows the 2 most common locations for augmentation: Behind the breast tissue, or subglandular (left image), and behind the pectoralis major, or subpectoral (right image).

Key Facts
- Synonyms: Implants, cosmetic augmentation
- Definition: Silicone elastomer bags filled with saline
  - Most have valves through which saline is injected at time of implant operation
    - Optimize cosmetic appearance
  - Some saline implants are prefilled
- Classic imaging appearance
  - Mammography examination includes implant and implant-displaced images
  - Implants located either behind glandular tissue (subglandular) or between pectoralis major and minor muscles (subpectoral)
  - Implants typically bilateral
    - Equal in size
    - Smooth
    - Most have visible valves
    - May have visible folds
- FDA approved for augmentation and reconstruction
- Only non-silicone gel-filled implants may be used for augmentation
- Not considered lifetime products
- > 20% require revision surgery

Imaging Findings
~graphy Findings
          ~" ∩ and CC views include implant
                 ' MLO and CC views emphasize breast tissue
                    or subpectoral in location
                    ni-opaque

Implant Saline

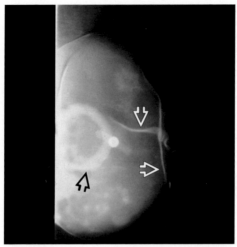

Implant saline view MLO mammogram shows both the valve (open black arrow) as well as folds of the silicone envelope (open white arrows). Despite the semi-transparent nature of the saline implant, the visualization of the breast tissue through the implant does not allow assessment of the obscured breast tissue.

- o Insufficient for assessing partially visible overlying breast tissue
- Implant folds and valves often seen
- Smooth or textured surface
- Encapsulation less common than with silicone implants
- Collapsed implants visible as ill-defined, dense regions
  - o The collapsed silicone envelope +/- body-made fibrous capsule
  - o Saline absorbed by body
  - o No residual visible material outside envelope/fibrous capsule

Ultrasound Findings
- No specific role
- Deflated saline implants will have little or no internal saline
- Extruded saline is absorbed

MR Findings
- No specific role for saline implant evaluation
- May be used to evaluate masses in women with prior history of silicone implants or injections
- May be helpful in assessing the implanted breast for occult malignancy
  - o Requires gadolinium injection
  - o Assessment of enhancing region(s) morphology and intensity

Differential Diagnosis
Silicone and Other Non-Saline Implants
- Opaque on mammogram
- Seldom allow visualization of folds or overlying obscured breast tissue

Pathology
General
- General Path Comments
  - o As foreign bodies, implants are walled off by body

- - Fibrous capsule
  - May be soft
  - May become very firm leading to varying degrees of encapsulation
  o Deflation rate reports vary greatly
    - 2-76%
    - Recent report = 8%

Gross Pathologic, Surgical Features
- Explanted material includes collapsed envelope
  o With or without fibrous capsule

Clinical Issues
Presentation
- Physical examination and patient issues are variable
  o Breast size
  o Implant location
  o Degree of encapsulation
  o Presence of implant rupture

Natural History
- Not a lifetime device
- Reported complications
  o Capsular contracture
  o Leakage
  o Rupture
  o Loss of nipple sensation
  o Asymmetry
  o Wrinkling or puckering of skin at implant sites

Treatment
- Symptomatic
- Ruptured implants are typically surgically removed
- Report of iatrogenic deflation of a saline implant following spontaneous rupture of the contralateral device without explantation

Prognosis
- No known association with breast cancer or collagen vascular disease
  o Careful attention to mammography and clinical examination to avoid missed cancers
    - Implant and implant-displaced views
    - Additional imaging evaluation with ultrasound and MRI not necessary for saline implant; helpful for workup of suspicious breast lesions

Selected References
1. Kinder EA et al: Iatrogenic intentional deflation of a saline breast implant after contralateral spontaneous implant deflation: A case report. J women's Imaging 4:179-81, 2002
2. Cunningham BL et al: Saline-filled breast implant safety and efficacy: A multicenter retrospective review. Plast & Recon surg 105:2143-9, 2000
3. Rohrich RJ: The FDA approves saline-filled breast implants: What does this mean for our patients? Plast and Recon Surg 106:903-5, 2000

Implant Silicone

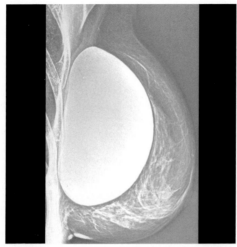

Implant silicone. Xerogram demonstrates relationship of a subglandular implant with the chest wall. No longer routinely used, this imaging method included the chest wall while film-screen mammography does not.

Key Facts
- Synonyms: Implants, post mastectomy reconstruction, cosmetic augmentation
- Definition: Breast size augmentation with surgically placed silicone gel contained within a silicone elastomer envelope
- Classic imaging appearance
  - Radiopaque, smooth oval prostheses in posterior breast
  - Implant displaced views allow visualization of most breast tissue
- FDA restricted silicone implant use in 1992
  - Post-mastectomy reconstruction or other medical indications
  - Not used for elective augmentation
- Medical concern with association of silicone & connective tissue disorders
  - American College of Rheumatology 1992
    - No convincing evidence that implants cause generalized disease
- Semipermeable nature of envelope may allow gel bleed
  - A difficult imaging diagnosis
- Not lifetime medical devices

Imaging Findings
General Features
- Placement = subglandular or between pectoralis major and minor
  - Implant-displaced views easier with subpectoral location
- Features often determined by implant type
  - Single or multiple lumen
  - With and without saline covering
  - Smooth or textured envelopes
- Non-encapsulated shape = oval
- Fibrous capsule forms around implant
  - Capsule may calcify
  - May be mammographically visible following explantation

Implant Silicone

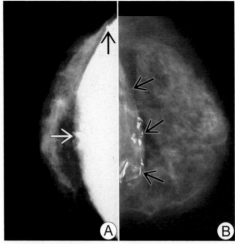

Implant silicone. (A) Coarse dystrophic calcifications (arrows) are visible within the fibrous capsule surrounding a silicone implant. (B) Patient status post explantation of a silicone implant with residual calcified fibrous capsule (arrows) clearly visible.

Mammography Findings
- Standard MLO & CC views designed to include a portion of implant
- Additional standard implant-displaced views "bleed" tissue away from implant allowing compression and visualization of breast tissue
- Additional diagnostic images performed as necessary
- Calcifications form in fibrous capsule
  - Parallel to implant surface
  - Sheet-like dystrophic characteristics
  - More common in subglandular than subpectoral location
- Shape changes associated with encapsulation
  - Baker's classification (I-IV) = a clinical assessment
  - Typically associated with fibrous capsule calcifications
  - Implant may be more rounded as encapsulation worsens
- Implant wrinkles
  - Likely to be as common as with saline implants
  - Silicone density limits visibility on mammography
- Report: Digital imaging may allow at least equal assessment of augmented breasts

Ultrasound Findings
- Intact implant is anechoic
  - Reverberation echo along anterior margin is normal
    - Should be no thicker than overlying breast tissue
- Breast mass evaluation is not limited by implant
- Knowledge of implant type may help in distinguishing possible rupture
  - Single, double, multiple lumen

MR Findings
- IR-FSE allows differentiation of silicone
  - Water + silicone – fat
  - Silicone – fat – water

Implant Silicone

- Fluid around implant does not mean rupture
- Folds or wrinkles in implant shell are common
  - Bright signal of silicone within folds = subtle sign intracapsular rupture
- Knowledge of implant type important to avoid misdiagnosis of rupture
- Positioning on breast coil may thin out medial implant simulating rupture
  - So-called "rat-tail" appearance

Imaging Recommendations
- Correlate clinical findings to be certain that areas of concern are included on implant and/or implant-displaced mammographic views
  - Despite the additional standard implant-displaced views, some breast tissue may be obscured
    - Hinders cancer detection
- Any concerning clinical finding should be evaluated

Differential Diagnosis
Implant Intracapsular Rupture
- May be asymptomatic with normal mammogram

Pathology
General
- Complications
  - Infection
  - Capsular contracture
  - Implant rupture
  - Possible systemic complications
    - Rheumatologic
    - Neurologic

Gross Pathologic, Surgical Features
- Explanted material may include fibrous capsule

Clinical Issues
Natural History
- The longer implants in place the greater potential for complications
  - Capsular contracture
  - Leakage
  - Rupture
  - Loss of nipple sensation
  - Puckering of skin at implant site

Treatment
- Complication-specific treatment as necessary

Prognosis
- No proven association with generalized collagen vascular disease
- No proven association with breast cancer

Selected References
1. Berg WA et al: MR imaging of extracapsular silicone from breast implants. AJR 178:465-72, 2002
2. Dickmann S et al: Digital full field mammography after breast augmentation. Radiology 42:275-9, 2002
3. Muzaffar AR et al: The silicone gel-filled breast implant controversy: An update. Plast and recon Surg 109:742-8, 2002

Implant Rupture

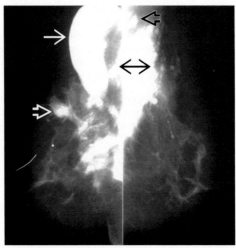

Implant rupture. Bilateral silicone implant extracapsular rupture and surgical explantation. Despite attempts at removal, residual silicone is seen as a focal mass (open white arrow), large areas of density (double headed arrow), a tubular density (white arrow) and lymph nodes (open black arrow).

Key Facts
- Definition: Rending of implant envelopes with extrusion of silicone or saline
  - Silicone may be contained by body made fibrous capsule
    - Intracapsular rupture
  - Silicone may be outside of fibrous capsule
    - Extracapsular rupture
- Classic imaging appearance
  - Collapse of silicone envelope of ruptured saline implant
    - Body resorbs saline
  - Extracapsular silicone implant rupture
    - Free silicone in breast tissue
  - Intracapsular silicone implant rupture
    - Mammogram may be negative
    - MRI best imaging modality
- Other key facts
  - Rupture may be asymptomatic
  - Implants are not lifetime medical devices
  - Incidental asymptomatic rupture = 6% or greater

Imaging Findings
Mammography Findings
- Extracapsular rupture with free silicone
  - Dense lobular or spherical areas of opacity
  - Linear deposits within lymphatics or along Cooper's ligaments
  - Droplets within lymph nodes
  - Dense masses may be silicone granulomas or "siliconomas"
  - Fibrosis
  - Silicone migration
- Intracapsular rupture

Implant Rupture

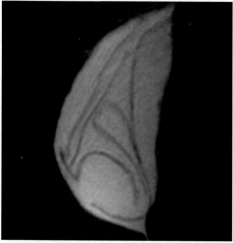

Implant rupture. Intracapsular silicone implant rupture. Sagittal MRI image shows numerous low intensity curvilinear lines representing the collapsed envelope floating in silicone held in place by the intact fibrous capsule. This is the so-called "linguine" sign.

- o Typically not helpful
- o Nonspecific findings may include herniation

Ultrasound Findings
- Extracapsular silicone may = "snowstorm"
  - o Increased echogenicity with loss of posterior detail
    - ▪ May see acoustic shadowing
  - o Large silicone granulomas or "siliconomas" = hypoechoic masses
    - ▪ May be surrounded by echogenic noise
- Intracapsular rupture findings
  - o Limited value
  - o Echogenic lines = collapsed envelope
    - ▪ "Step-ladder" sign
  - o Debris or diffuse low level internal echoes
  - o Decrease in anteroposterior (A-P) implant dimension

MR Findings
- Not required for evaluation of saline implant rupture
- Free silicone = discrete low signal intensity foci on fat-suppressed T1
  - o High signal intensity on water suppressed T2
- Pulse sequences specific for demonstrating silicone are available
- Intracapsular findings
  - o Collapsed shell surrounded by silicone = "linguine" sign
  - o Subtle signs = small amounts of extruded silicone
    - ▪ Collections on implant shell surface = subcapsular line sign
    - ▪ Collections within implant shell folds = "keyhole" or "noose" signs
    - ▪ Suggest implant shell failure or "uncollapsed rupture"

Imaging Recommendations
- When rupture suspected, MRI most helpful - sensitivity 72-94%; specialty 85-100%

Implant Rupture

Differential Diagnosis
Masses
- Silicone granuloma may be indistinguishable from other hypoechoic masses such as carcinoma
- Biopsy may be required to differentiate

Pathology
General
- Rupture sequela
  - Gel migration
    - Local and distant
    - Reported to drain through fistulas and cause skin ulceration
  - Inflammation
  - Silicone granuloma formation
Microscopic Features
- Non-contained silicone local adverse effects
  - Fibrosis
  - Granuloma formation
    - Empty vacuoles = free silicone
    - Foreign-body giant cells

Clinical Issues
Presentation
- Ruptured silicone should be asymptomatic
- Complaints related to rupture
  - Change in breast size; pain
  - Masses (breast, axilla, chest wall)
  - Intraductal extension
    - Nipple discharge of silicone gel
  - Silicone migration into brachial plexus may = neuropathy
- Rupture attributed to closed capsulotomy
  - External manipulation of encapsulated implants
  - Not a common practice today
- Rupture attributed to mammography described as a popping sound
  - Believed related to rupture of fibrous capsule
Natural History
- Implants are not lifetime devices
Treatment
- Ruptured implants may be explanted
- Challenging to remove all of free silicone
Prognosis
- No proven association with generalized collagen vascular disease
- No proven association with breast cancer

Selected References
1. Contant CM et al: A prospective study of silicone breast implants and the silicone-related symptom complex. Clin Rheumatol 21:215-9, 2002
2. Middleton MS et al: Breast implant classification with MR imaging correlation. Radiographics 20:E1, 2000
3. Caskey CI et al: Imaging spectrum of extrascpaular silicone: Correlation of US, MR imaging, mammographic, and histopathologic findings. Radiographics 19:S39-51, 1999

Reduction Mammaplasty

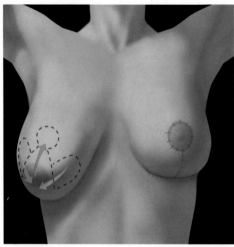

Reduction mammoplasty. The right breast portion of the diagram demonstrates the surgical approach used for the "keyhole" surgical incision technique where the nipple and ducts are left attached. The post-surgical appearance is presented on the left breast image.

Key Facts
- Synonyms: Breast reduction, breast reconstruction, reduction surgery
- Definition: Breast tissue removal to reduce size of breast
- Classic imaging appearance
  - Parenchyma redistributed from upper to lower breast
- Keyhole surgical incision technique (most common)
  - Incision along inframammary fold & vertical incision along 6 o'clock to nipple
  - Tissue in lower breast resected
    - Remaining tissue moves from a high to low position
  - Nipple/areolar complex repositioning no matter how procedure is performed
  - Nipple attached to ducts in pedicle flap with dermal transposition
    - Preserves breast feeding ability
    - Nipple sensation generally preserved
  - Alternative method = pedicle flaps with full-thickness nipple areolar graft
    - Ducts are severed from the nipple
  - Redundant skin removed & lower incisions pulled together

Imaging Findings
General Features
- Best imaging clue
  - Parenchyma redistributed from upper to lower breast
  - Nipple elevated
Mammography Findings
- Variable findings
  - From no significant abnormality to pronounced architectural distortion
  - Findings determined by surgical technique
- Swirling configuration of remolded tissue

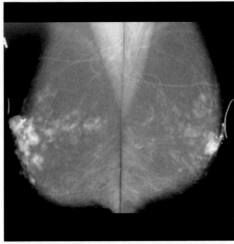

Reduction mammoplasty. 54-year-old woman following reduction mammoplasty. MLO views from the mammogram demonstrate elevation of the nipples, patchy redistribution of tissue, relocation of most of the tissue at or below the nipple line, and coarse calcifications c/w fat necrosis in the retroareolar regions.

- o Parenchyma redistributed from upper to lower breast
- Elevation of nipple
- Nonanatomic scars and parenchymal bands
  - o Areas of scarring regress over time
- Fat necrosis (20%)
  - o Lipid oil cyst (calcified or uncalcified)
  - o Clustered microcalcifications
    - ▪ Often located in retroareolar region
    - ▪ Likely secondary to nipple/areolar repositioning
  - o Spiculated area of increased opacity
  - o Focal mass
  - o May mimic malignancy
- Dystrophic benign calcifications
  - o Usually occur several years following surgery
  - o May develop in parenchyma &/or skin
- Skin thickening

Imaging Recommendations
- Baseline mammogram performed prior to procedure
  - o To detect occult carcinoma
- Postoperative mammogram performed at 6 months for new baseline
  - o Variable – based on patient age

Differential Diagnosis
Carcinoma
- May be indistinguishable from scar & fat necrosis

Pathology
General
- General Path Comments

Reduction Mammaplasty

- o Excised tissue from reduction should be sent for pathologic analysis
- • Etiology-Pathogenesis
  - o Epithelial inclusion cyst may occur (rare)
- • Epidemiology
  - o More common in obese patients

Clinical Issues
Presentation
- • Indications for macromastia
  - o Cosmesis/self-image
  - o Physical disability
- • To match mastectomy with contralateral reconstruction
- • Gigantomastia of pregnancy (rare)

Natural History
- • May present with palpable abnormality after reduction
  - o Fat necrosis
  - o Hematoma
  - o Scar
- • Any palpable mass following reduction evaluated in usual manner
  - o Tissue sampling may be warranted

Treatment
- • None

Prognosis
- • High patient satisfaction following procedure

Selected References
1. Mitnick JS et al: Distinction between postsurgical changes and carcinoma by means of stereotaxic fine-needle aspiration biopsy after reduction mammaplasty. Radiology 188:457-62, 1993
2. Mendelson EB: Evaluation of the postoperative breast. Radiol Clin North Am 30:107-38, 1992
3. Miller CL et al: Mammographic changes after reduction mammoplasty. AJR 149:35-8, 1987

PocketRadiologist®
Breast
Top 100 Diagnoses

POST-OP CANCER

Edema & Breast Conservation

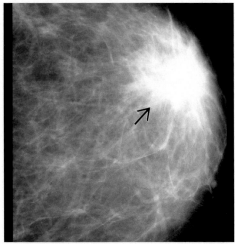

Edema & breast conservation. Mammogram of postoperative edema involving the entire breast. Lumpectomy site is shown as spiculated mass (arrow).

Key Facts
- Synonyms: Lymphedema, postsurgical changes, post-therapy changes
- Definition: Presence of abnormally large amounts of fluid in intercellular tissue spaces of breast
- Classic imaging appearance: Increased mammographic density due to skin and trabecular thickening
- General causes of edema
  - Lymphatic or venous obstruction
  - Increased vascular permeability
  - Systemic
- Sequelae of breast conserving therapy (BCT)
- Severity not related to radiation dose (RT)
- Arm lymphedema more likely in full axillary dissection (10-20%)
  - Serious debilitating swelling that adversely affects quality of life
- Sentinel lymph node biopsy lowers rate of lymphedema (1-2%)

Imaging Findings
General Features
- Best imaging clue: Diffuse density & distortion; skin and trabecular thickening

Mammography Findings
- Post treatment edema
  - Skin & trabecular thickening
  - Diffuse increased density & distortion
- Maximum changes on first mammogram at 6 months post RT
  - Findings diminish on subsequent examinations
  - Usually improve/resolve by 1–3 yrs
- Increasing edema may be due to recurrent cancer

Ultrasound Findings
- Skin thickening, parenchymal echogenicity changes, dilated lymphatic channels

Edema & Breast Conservation

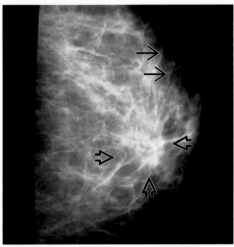

Edema & breast conservation. Mammogram of postoperative edema showing thickening of trabeculae (arrows) and skin thickening. Lumpectomy site (open arrows) in this example not as prominent.

<u>T1 C+ MR Findings</u>
- Postradiation skin & parenchymal enhancement can occur for many yrs following treatment (variable)

<u>Imaging Recommendations</u>
- Baseline mammography recommended 6 months after end of RT
- Surgical scar must be fully included on mammogram
- Annual mammogram thereafter

Differential Diagnosis
<u>Inflammatory Breast Cancer Recurrence</u>
- Skin biopsy differentiates cases where resolution of edema prolonged
  - Tumor emboli seen in dermal lymphatics

<u>Lymphedema Due To Nodal Recurrence</u>
<u>Venous Congestion</u>
- Congestive heart failure/mediastinal or axillary masses

<u>Lymphoma</u>
<u>Mastitis</u>
- Clinical features include fever, redness, tenderness

Pathology
<u>General</u>
- General Path Comments
  - Lymphedema occurs when lymphatic transport capacity exceeded
  - Buildup of interstitial molecules increases oncotic pressure
    - Leads to more edema
  - Radiation causes vascular changes
    - Small vessel wall necrosis
    - Narrowing/obliteration of arterial lumens

Edema & Breast Conservation

- Etiology-Pathogenesis
  - o Engorgement of the dermal and intramammary lymphatics
    - Results in trabecular thickening
  - o Postradiation edema thought to be in response to inflammation
- Epidemiology
  - o More common in obese patients

Microscopic Features
- Radiation changes
  - o Atypical epithelial cells in the terminal ductal lobular unit (TDLU)
  - o Lobular sclerosis and atrophy

Clinical Issues

Presentation
- Seen in early post-treatment phase
- Skin erythema may accompany edema
- Skin thickening > 3-4 mm is unusual for radiation alone
- Arm lymphedema results in swelling, numbness & pain

Natural History
- Chronic edema may progress to permanent skin fibrosis
  - o Mammographic pattern indistinguishable from acute edema
  - o Increased risk in scleroderma (contraindication to RT) & rheumatoid arthritis (relative contraindication to RT)
- Arm lymphedema
  - o Predisposed to cellulitis & lymphangitis

Treatment
- None if limited to breast
- If associated with lymphedema of arm, treatment advised
  - o Compression garments, massage, physiotherapy
  - o Microsurgery may be advised
    - More helpful earlier before fibrosis occurs

Prognosis
- Transient phenomenon
  - o Usually resolves after 1-3 years (widely variable)
- May take prolonged period to resolve
  - o Development of collateral lymphatic drainage needed

Selected References
1. Dershaw DD: Mammography in patients with breast cancer treated by breast conservation (lumpectomy with or without radiation). AJR 164(2):309-16, 1995
2. Mendelson EB: Evaluation of the postoperative breast. Radiol Clin North Am 30:107-38, 1992
3. Pezner RD et al: Breast edema in patients treated conservatively for stage I and II breast cancer. Int J Radiat Oncol Biol Phys 11(10):1765-8, 1985

Post-Mastectomy Reconstruction

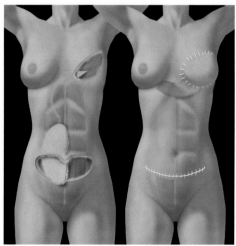

Post-mastectomy reconstruction. Drawing illustrates the pedicled TRAM operation.

Key Facts
- Definition: Restoration to closely resemble anatomic form and characteristics of normal breast following mastectomy
  - Exogenous implant reconstruction (silicone or saline)
  - Autologous vascularized flap reconstruction
- Typical mammographic appearance
  - Exogenous implant: Radiodense implant with overlying tissues
  - Flap reconstructions: Breast-like mammographic appearance, asymmetric usually radiolucent fatty appearance
- Other key facts
  - Controversy over need for any surveillance imaging
  - Recurrent malignancy
    - Imaging may detect before clinical examination
    - Most recurrences are invasive carcinoma in cases of prior multifocal ductal carcinoma in situ (DCIS)

Imaging Findings
Mammography Findings
- Implant reconstruction
  - Radiodense implant, no overlying breast parenchyma
  - Additional views (lateromedial) if implant cannot be displaced
  - Implant deformity suggests capsular herniation, intracapsular rupture
- Flap reconstruction
  - Common findings
    - Dense "glandular cone" (if muscle), or mainly fatty density
    - Curvilinear fibrous densities
    - Dystrophic calcifications
    - Fat necrosis (calcifications +/- focal irregular density)
Ultrasound Findings
- Color Doppler useful for preoperative pedicle artery mapping

Post-Mastectomy Reconstruction

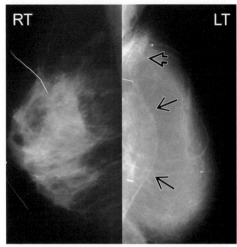

MLO views of a 63-year-old woman 4 years after TRAM flap reconstruction of left breast. The muscle flap is the soft tissue (arrows) against the chest wall in the otherwise totally fatty reconstructed left breast. Vague soft tissue superior density (open arrow) is from recent benign biopsy for new calcifications.

- Limited role in surveillance
- Characterize focal mammographic abnormality (e.g., mass)
- May detect intracapsular silicone implant rupture
- Can be used to guide needle biopsy of focal lesions

MR Findings
- Limited role in surveillance
- Can characterize focal abnormality
- Best for detection of intracapsular silicone implant rupture ("linguine" sign)
- Can detect tumor recurrence behind implant if subcutaneous

Imaging Recommendations
- Mammographic surveillance
  - Depends on institution
  - Perhaps for multifocal DCIS cases with reconstruction
- Ultrasound for lesion characterization, needle biopsy
- MRI may be helpful occasionally, especially if implants present

Differential Diagnosis
Recurrent Cancer vs Post-Procedural Complication/Finding
- Any change in physical exam or imaging must be evaluated

Pathology
- No specific findings

Clinical Issues
Implant Reconstruction
- Delayed reconstruction usually
- Tissue expanders initially implanted
- Retropectoral or subcutaneous implant (silicone or saline)

Post-Mastectomy Reconstruction

Myocutaneous Flaps
- Immediate or delayed reconstruction
- Deep inferior epigastric pedicle flap
  - Skin & fat only, bilateral deep inferior epigastric artery pedicles
  - Rectus preserved, no tunnel, flap can be split for bilateral use

Pedicled or Free Transverse Rectus Abdominis Myocutaneous (TRAM) Flap
- Large transverse ellipse from lower abdomen
- Deep superior epigastric artery (DSEA) supplies rectus abdominis

Contralateral Rectus Abdominis, Fascia & Overlying Skin Mobilized
- Pedicled TRAM: Flap with DSEA pedicle rotated 90-180° with subcutaneous tunnel to mastectomy site (may leave bulge)
- Free TRAM: Flap and DSEA excised, anastomosed to axillary or internal mammary vessels (no tunnel or bulge)
- Fascial and rectus defect sutured or repaired with mesh

Other Flaps (Uncommon)
- Latissimus dorsi (axillary incision)
- Gluteal (free pedicle flap)

Main Complications
- Implant reconstruction
  - Delayed implant rupture
  - Capsular contracture
- Myocutaneous flap reconstruction
  - Abdominal hernia (TRAM only)
  - Flap necrosis or infection (scar, marked deformity)
  - Donor site necrosis or infection (scarring)
  - Fat necrosis (calcifications, irregular mass)

Examination
- Breast symmetry often excellent (especially myocutaneous flaps)
- May have palpable thickening, deformity

Natural History
- Recurrent tumor quite uncommon (< 2% within 2 years)
- Delayed implant rupture quite common (> 50% at 10 years)

Treatment
- That of underlying pathology

Prognosis
- That of underlying pathology

Controversy Over Surveillance Imaging
- No evidence of improved survival if recurrent cancer detected
  - By imaging (mammography)
  - By clinical palpation
- But increased risk of recurrence if extensive DCIS with close margins
  - Usually invasive ductal carcinoma at time of detection
  - This category may warrant mammographic surveillance
- Practice varies widely
- Institutional consensus recommended

Selected References
1. Helvie MA et al: Mammographic screening of TRAM flap breast reconstructions for detection of nonpalpable recurrent cancer. Radiology 224:211-6, 2002
2. Herborn CU et al: Breast augmentation and reconstructive surgery: MR imaging of implant rupture and malignancy. Eur Radiol 12:2198-206, 2002
3. Giunta RE et al: The value of preoperative Doppler sonography for planning free perforator flaps. Plast Reconstr Surg 105:2381-6, 2000

Post-Op Calcifications

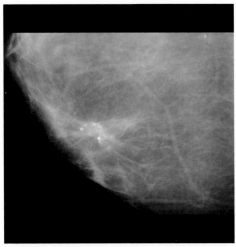

Post-op calcifications. Magnification view of a mammogram showing benign calcifications compatible with fat necrosis at lumpectomy site. Note lucent centers and curvilinear calcifications.

Key Facts
- Definition: Benign calcifications that form after breast conserving treatment (BCT) including lumpectomy & radiation therapy (RT)
- Classic imaging appearance: Lucent centered, coarse, spherical, ovoid calcifications (Ca++)
- Types of (Ca++)
  - o Fat necrosis
  - o Dystrophic
  - o Sutural
  - o Calcifications related to cancer recurrence
- Early stage of benign Ca++ may mimic breast cancer recurrence
  - o Distinguish by biopsy
  - o Assessment by BIRADS criteria for biopsy
- Benign Ca++ after benign breast biopsy are uncommon
  - o The major insult to breast is not biopsy, but RT used in breast conserving treatment
- Sutural Ca++ related to
  - o Extensive surgery (reduction mammoplasty)
  - o Delayed healing after RT
- Benign calcifications after RT
  - o 33% of irradiated breasts develop Ca++ 2–3 yrs after RT
    - ▪ 50% sutural
    - ▪ Can develop up to 4 yrs after RT
  - o Due to combination of trauma from surgery & RT
  - o Large, irregular with central lucency
  - o Occur at surgical site

Imaging Findings
<u>General Features</u>
- Best imaging clue: Coarse, lucent-centered, ovoid, spherical Ca++

Post-Op Calcifications

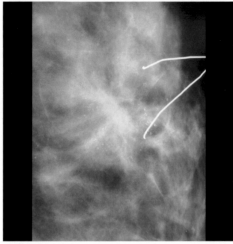

Mammogram magnification view of 60-year-old, 5 years after lumpectomy & RT. Scattered pleomorphic calcifications are at the lumpectomy site. Stereotactic biopsy demonstrated recurrent infiltrating ductal carcinoma. Patient underwent mastectomy.

<u>Mammography Findings</u>
- Fat necrosis
  - Calcified or non-calcified oil cysts
  - +/- Spiculated/focal irregular mass
  - Early Ca++ may mimic recurrence
- Dystrophic
  - Lucent-centered, coarse, ovoid
- Recurrence
  - Recurrence at lumpectomy site rare in first 2 yrs
  - Minority of recurrences contain calcifications
  - Biopsy Ca++ classified as BIRADS 4 or 5

<u>Ultrasound Findings</u>
- Ca++ not reliably seen

<u>Post C+ T1 MR Findings</u>
- Ca++ not reliably seen

<u>Imaging Recommendations</u>
- Conventional & magnifications views for suspicious Ca++
- First post-surgical mammogram obtained at 6 months to 1 yr
- Recurrence within 18 mos after RT unusual if surgical margins free from tumor at the time of lumpectomy
  - Specimen radiograph/post-operative mammogram documents removal of mammographic lesion
  - Final pathology confirms lesion size, grade, and margin status

Differential Diagnosis
<u>None</u>

Post-Op Calcifications

Pathology

General

- General Path Comments
  - Hemosiderin-laden macrophages may mimic Ca++
    - No imaging characteristics specific enough to differentiate
    - Suspicious findings must be biopsied
- Etiology-Pathogenesis
  - Fat necrosis develops due to benign suppurative process
  - Sutural Ca++ pathogenesis unknown
- Epidemiology
  - 25-35% patients develop benign Ca++ after BCT

Clinical Issues

Presentation

- Mammographic presentation

Treatment

- None for benign Ca++
- Any suspicious finding must be evaluated and biopsied
- Recurrent carcinoma generally requires mastectomy

Prognosis

- Good for benign Ca++

Selected References

1. Dershaw DD: Evaluation of the breast undergoing lumpectomy and radiation therapy. Radiol Clin N Am 33:1147-60; 1995
2. Hogge JP, et al: The mammographic spectrum of fat necrosis of the breast. Radiolgraphics 15(6):1347-56; 1995
3. DPhil DY, et al: A mammographic dilemma: calcification or haemosiderin as a cause of opacities? Validation of a new digital diagnostic tool. British J of Radiology 74:1048-51, 2001

Post Surgical Seromas And Scars

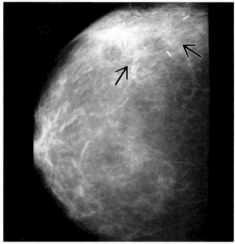

Mammogram of postoperative distortion after lumpectomy (arrows). Note the diffuse increased density and trabecular coarsening (edema) of the breast as well as the clips marking the lumpectomy site.

Key Facts
- Synonyms: Post-biopsy changes, Post-biopsy hematoma
- Definition
  - Seroma: Serous fluid collection in dead space of biopsy cavity
  - Hematoma: Active bleeding at surgical site forms a collection
  - Scar: Dense fibrous tissue with surrounding retraction
- Classic imaging appearance
  - Seroma & hematoma usually indistinguishable
    - Radiodense, oval, ill-defined, dense mass
    - Occupies the surgical cavity
  - Scar
    - Architectural distortion
    - Spiculated elongated mass
- Seroma/hematoma usually resorbed completely or becomes a scar
- Seroma/hematoma may become chronic & may calcify

Imaging Findings
Mammography Findings
- Abnormal mammograms after biopsy 50%
- Seroma/hematoma
  - Oval, dense, ill-defined mass
  - Acutely may see air/fluid level
  - Becomes more demarcated with increasing age
- Scar
  - Architectural distortion or spiculated mass
    - Verify that finding corresponds to surgical site
    - Place wire skin marker over cutaneous scar before mammogram
  - Looks worse on one view
  - Fat is often seen centrally
  - Size and density should decrease over time

Post Surgical Seromas And Scars

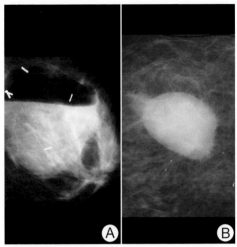

Examples of seromas/hematomas on mammography. (A) Mammogram of acute seroma with air-fluid level. (B) Chronic hematoma shows partial calcification. This finding had been stable for 5 yrs.

- o Difficult to distinguish from malignancy
- Associated post RT stromal coarsening and skin thickening
  - o May obscure surgical site on initial mammogram
- Associated reactive axillary adenopathy may be present

Ultrasound Findings
- Hematoma
  - o Hypoechoic irregular cystic mass with echogenic components
    - ▪ Clots/fibrinous debris
  - o With increase in age, more defined borders
- Seroma
  - o Presents like hematoma with less echogenicity
  - o Ultrasound guidance may be used to outline post-lumpectomy seroma for radiation therapy boost planning (following whole breast irradiation)
- Scar
  - o Hypoechoic linear lesion that extends to skin

T1 C+ MR Imaging
- Acute seroma/hematoma
  - o Low to high signal intensity cavity depending on age
  - o Thin (< 5 mm) peripheral enhancement from granulation tissue
- Subacute/chronic seroma/hematoma
  - o Irregular, spiculated mass
  - o Suspicious morphology & kinetics
- Scar
  - o Thin linear enhancement
  - o May enhance years following surgery
- Useful to assess residual bulky disease after surgery with positive margins

Imaging Recommendations
- Baseline mammogram obtained at 6 months following RT
- Surgical site must be fully imaged
  - o For future comparison

Post Surgical Seromas And Scars

- All scars should be marked on a clinical diagram of the breast
  - For interpretation of mammographic findings
- For confirmation of scar
  - Compare with preoperative films for location of surgery
  - Place wire marker for mammogram & do cone views if necessary
  - Correlate with physical examination

Differential Diagnosis
Invasive Carcinoma
- Difficult to distinguish from scar
- Biopsy indicated if cannot confirm scar
Recurrent Carcinoma
- Increased prominence of the scar over time raises suspicion

Pathology
General
- Etiology-Pathogenesis
  - Hematoma develops from frank bleeding at operative site
  - Seroma develops from collection of serous fluid
  - Scar develops after collections have resorbed
    - More likely to develop scar following hematoma
- Epidemiology
  - Post surgical hematoma requiring drainage 0.5-4%
    - Inadequate hemostasis
    - Altered platelet function or bleeding disorders

Clinical Issues
Presentation
- Mammographic finding
Natural History
- Mammographic findings should decrease over time
  - May stabilize or resolve
Treatment
- Drainage of postoperative seroma/hematoma if
  - Infected
  - Large & palpable, obscuring physical examination
  - Painful
Prognosis
- Good

Selected References
1. Krishnamurthy R et al: Mammographic findings after breast conservation therapy. Radiographics 19 Spec No:S53-62, 1999
2. Birdwell RL, et al. Sonographic tailoring of electron beam boost site after lumpectomy and radiation therapy for breast cancer. AJR 168:39-40, 1997
3. Dershaw DD: Mammography in patients with breast cancer treated by breast conservation (lumpectomy with or without radiation). AJR 164:309-16, 1995

Recurrent Breast Carcinoma

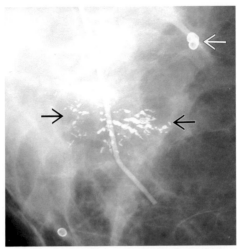

Recurrent breast carcinoma. Spot magnification mammogram of patient 1 year following breast conservation therapy for high-grade DCIS. (Note linear scar marker) Reveals new linear branching calcifications (BIRADS 5) that represent recurrent high-grade DCIS (black arrows). Benign fat necrosis calcifications (white arrow).

Key Facts
- Synonym: Local recurrence
- Definition: Appearance of carcinoma at lumpectomy site or elsewhere in breast following breast conservation therapy
- Recurrence diagnosed by mammography 35-50%
- More likely to detect noninvasive recurrence by mammography
  - Ductal carcinoma in situ (DCIS) seen as calcifications
- Less likely to detect invasive noncalcified recurrence by mammography
  - Invasive carcinoma seen as noncalcified mass
- Histology of recurrence is invasive in majority

Imaging Findings
General Features
- Best imaging clue: New calcifications or mass at lumpectomy site or elsewhere in treated breast
Mammography Findings
- Detects recurrence in 35-50%
- Physical examination detects majority (67%)
- New suspicious microcalcifications
- Ill-defined, increasing density/mass
Ultrasound Findings
- Mass at lumpectomy site
  - Benign scar may shadow
  - Able to see extension to skin surface
- Post-operative hematoma/seroma common 6-12+ months post-op
  - If radiation used
  - Resolves sooner if no radiation therapy
MR Findings
- T1 C+

Recurrent Breast Carcinoma

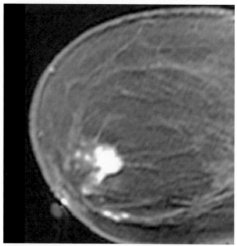

Recurrent breast carcinoma, T1 C+ MR. Patient with new palpable fullness at the lumpectomy site. Mammography revealed post-operative scarring & density but no suspicious calcifications. T1 C+ MR shows an irregular enhancing mass at lumpectomy site (skin marker), indicating recurrent invasive ductal carcinoma.

- o Nodular enhancement if recurrent invasive
- o Linear enhancement seen with DCIS and scar
- o Scar may enhance up to 18 months post surgery

Imaging Recommendations
- Magnification views to assess new calcifications at lumpectomy site
- Rolled views if new mass suspected
- Ultrasound if mammogram inconclusive for presence of mass
- MR if ultrasound inconclusive

Differential Diagnosis
Fat Necrosis
- Late coarse calcifications usually easy to discriminate
- Early fat necrosis calcifications can mimic recurrence

Scar
- Appears different and less dense on orthogonal views
- May disappear on rolled views
- Remains stable or decreases in density and size over time

Pathology
General
- General Path Comments
  - o Completeness of excision of a breast cancer impacts on risk of recurrence
    - Negative inked margins decrease chance of recurrence
  - o Pathology of recurrences
    - Infiltrating carcinoma (50%) & DCIS (50%)
- Etiology-Pathogenesis
  - o Untreated disease at or close to lumpectomy site usually appears within 2 years

- o New breast primary arises elsewhere in breast after 2 years

Clinical Issues

Presentation
- Palpable mass at lumpectomy site in 67%
- Following at increased risk for recurrence
  - o Extensive intraductal component (> 25% of tumor microscopically) associated with infiltrating ductal carcinoma
  - o Young age (< 40 years)
  - o Estrogen receptor negative
  - o Positive margins
  - o DCIS > 2-5 cm (more likely multicentric)
  - o Comedo type DCIS
  - o Lymphatic invasion

Natural History
- 1–2% per year
- Recurrence < 18 months rare if optimal treatment administered
- Carcinoma 4-6 years after therapy = local failure
  - o Usually occurs at or near lumpectomy site
- Carcinoma > 6 years following therapy = new primary
  - o Usually away from lumpectomy site

Treatment
- Mastectomy if patient has already received radiation therapy
- Consideration for re-excision if patient has not received radiation therapy
  - o Controversial treatment option

Prognosis
- Long-term disease-free survival equal to that of breast conservation (30-50%)
- Concurrent metastatic disease in 5-10%
- Locally extensive recurrences in 5-10% (poorer prognosis)
- Tumors > 2 cm at recurrence and diffuse dermal involvement have poorer prognosis
- Longer the time to recurrence the better the prognosis

Selected References
1. Dershaw DD: Breast imaging and the conservative treatment of breast cancer. Radiol Clin North Am 40(3):501-16, 2002
2. Rodrigues N: Correlation of clinical and pathologic features with outcome in patients with ductal carcinoma in situ of the breast treated with breast-conserving surgery and radiotherapy. Int J Radiat Oncol Biol Phys 54(5):1331-5, 2002
3. Greenstein S et al: Breast cancer recurrence after lumpectomy and irradiation: Role of mammography in detection. Radiology 183:201-6, 1992

PocketRadiologist®
Breast
Top 100 Diagnoses

HORMONE CHANGES

Hormone Replacement Therapy

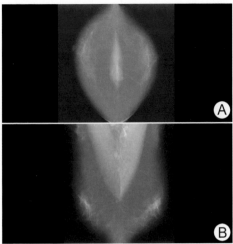

Hormone replacement therapy. 51-year-old asymptomatic woman before hormone replacemnet therapy. (A) Bilateral CC views. (B) Bilateral MLO views.

Key Facts
- Definition: Exogenous hormonal supplementation to offset declining levels of estrogen and progesterone in postmenopausal women
- Classic imaging appearance
  - Bilateral and symmetrical increase in breast density after institution of hormone replacement therapy (HRT)
- Route of administration
  - Oral
    - Most common
  - Skin patch
  - Intramuscular injection
- HRT reverses normal postmenopausal involutional processes
  - Proliferation of glandular and stromal elements
  - Cessation or reversal of progressive fatty replacement
- Useful for control of menopause symptoms
  - Hot flashes
  - Vaginal dryness
  - Insomnia
  - Night sweats
- Risks of combination (estrogen and progesterone) HRT
  - Results of Women's Health Initiative (WHI) controlled, prospective randomized trial
    - Increased risk invasive breast cancer 29%
    - No increased risk DCIS
    - Increased risk coronary heart disease, stroke and pulmonary emboli
- Health benefits
  - Osteoporosis prevention
    - 33% decrease in hip fractures

Hormone Replacement Therapy

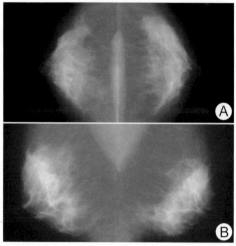

Hormone replacement therapy. Same case as previous page, one year after beginning hormone replacement therapy. Note bilateral and symmetrical increase in density. (A) Bilateral CC view. (B) Bilateral MLO view.

- 22% decrease other osseous fractures
  - o Colorectal cancer
    - 37% decrease

Imaging Findings
Mammography Findings
- Generalized increase in mammographic density
  - o Usually bilateral and symmetrical
  - o May be asymmetric and/or patchy
    - Must differentiate from evolving mass
    - Obtain additional views, ultrasound
  - o Density measured by two methods
    - Qualitative breast density assessment
    - Upward shift 24% in HRT patients
    - Quantitative density measurement
    - Increase 73% in HRT patients
  - o Most pronounced in patients with lower baseline density
  - o Density changes more common with combination HRT than estrogen alone
  - o Degree of density change not affected by duration of HRT
- Increase in breast size
- Proliferation of cysts and fibroadenomas in postmenopausal women
  - o More common with estrogen alone
- No statistically significant decrease in mammographic sensitivity in women on HRT
  - o Slight decrease in specificity
Ultrasound Findings
- Tissue stimulated by HRT usually homogeneous and hyperechoic
- May be normal

Hormone Replacement Therapy

- Helpful in cystic-solid differentiation of masses suspected to be caused by hormonal stimulation

Imaging Recommendations
- May recommend interval mammogram following cessation of HRT to evaluate for problem cases to rule out possible developing mass(es)
- MRI may be used at some institutions for problem cases

Differential Diagnosis

Pregnancy

Lactation

Bilateral Inflammatory Carcinoma (Extremely Rare)
- Associated with edema, erythema and peau d'orange

Pathology

General
- Estrogen effects
  - Normal breast epithelium stimulated to proliferate
    - Elongation of small terminal ducts
    - Lobule formation
  - Proliferation of stromal elements, interlobular connective tissue
- Progesterone effects
  - Increase in epithelial mitotic activity
  - Increased lobule size
  - Stromal edema

Clinical Issues

Presentation
- Breast pain
  - Occurs in 25% of women on HRT
  - Dose dependent
  - Associated with increase in mammographic density
- Prognosis
  - Increased risk of breast cancer in patients on HRT
    - More biologically favorable tumors in HRT users compared with non-users
    - Increased frequency of T1 lesions, node negative tumors and stage I tumors
    - More DCIS among users
    - Greatest risk among users on HRT ten or more years
    - HRT before cancer diagnosis may increase survival by as much as 13%

Selected References
1. Carney, PA: Individual and combined effects of age, breast density, and hormone replacement Therapy use on the accuracy of screening mammography. Annals Internal Medicine. 138(3):168-75, 2003
2. Roussouw, JE et al: Risks and benefits of estrogen plus progestin in healthy postmenopausal women: Principal results from the women's health initiative randomized controlled trial. JAMA 288(3):321-33, 2002
3. Thurfjell, EL et al: Screening mammography: Sensitivity and specificity in relation to hormone replacement therapy. Radiology 203:339-41, 1997

Malignancy and Pregnancy

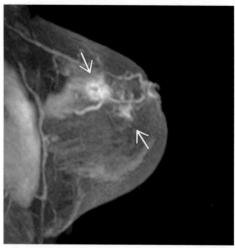

Malignancy and pregnancy. 38-year-old woman recent postpartum and lactating presents with palpable abnormality in upper outer quadrant followed for several months without resolution. Maximum intensity projection of a T1 C+ MR image demonstrates multicentric infiltrating ductal carcinoma (arrows).

Key Facts
- Synonym: Pregnancy-associated breast carcinoma
- Definition: Breast cancer during pregnancy or within 1 yr postpartum
- Classic imaging appearance: Identical to non-pregnancy-related carcinoma
- Diagnostic delay is common (1–6 months)
- No current evidence that carcinoma in pregnancy more aggressive

Imaging Findings
<u>General Features</u>
- Best imaging clue: Identical to non pregnancy related carcinoma
- Mammography may be falsely negative up to 35%
- Two view mammography (0.4 mrad to fetus)
  - Careful counseling with patient
  - Different risks depending on trimester

<u>Ultrasound Findings</u>
- Identical to non pregnancy related carcinoma

<u>MR Findings</u>
- T1 C+
  - Not recommended for first trimester
  - False positive enhancement from hormonal stimulation possible
  - Use of gadolinium in pregnancy not recommended
    - Unless potential risk to patient outweighs risk to fetus

<u>Imaging Recommendations</u>
- Ultrasound first test of choice
  - Can distinguish cyst from solid mass
- Mammography
  - Perform after nursing or pumping, if applicable
  - Shield abdomen with lead aprons if pregnant

Malignancy and Pregnancy

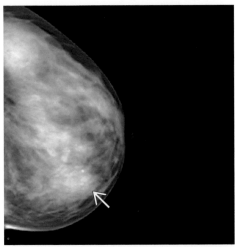

Malignancy and pregnancy. Mammogram. 37-year-old woman breast-feeding a newborn presents with palpable abnormality in upper outer quadrant. Mammogram demonstrates dense breast with benign calcifications (arrow) in lower inner quadrant. Palpable mass pathology yielded infiltrating ductal carcinoma.

Differential Diagnosis
Fibroadenoma
Lactating Adenoma
Lobular Hyperplasia
Galactocele
Abscess
Lipoma
Hamartoma
Leukemia, Lymphoma, Sarcoma, Neuroma, and Tuberculosis (Rare)

Pathology
General
- General Path Comments
  - Similar to non-pregnancy-related carcinoma
- Genetics
  - Genetic predisposition (BRCA 1 & 2) more prone
    - High levels of estrogen may accelerate malignancy
  - Family history of breast cancer also more common
- Epidemiology
  - Most common malignancy in pregnancy
  - 1:3,000–10,000 pregnancies
  - Incidence of inflammatory carcinoma similar to non pregnancy related carcinoma

Microscopic Features
- Histologically similar to non-pregnancy-related carcinoma
- More likely to be estrogen-receptor negative

Staging or Grading Criteria
- Generally occur at a later stage
  - Thought to be due to a delay in diagnosis

Malignancy and Pregnancy

- Compared with non-pregnancy-related carcinoma
  - Tumors are larger
  - More likely to have positive nodes (60-70%)
  - More likely to have metastases, and vascular invasion

Clinical Issues

Presentation
- Painless mass or thickening
- Nipple discharge
- If breast feeding, infant may refuse milk from breast

Natural History
- Recurrence rates high if pregnancy occurs immediately after treatment
  - 50% 5-yr survival – pregnancy within 1 year
  - 83% 5-yr survival – pregnancy 1–2 years
  - 100% 5-yr survival – pregnancy after 2 years
- Limited experience with subsequent pregnancy following breast carcinoma
  - In general, future pregnancy not advised for
    - Positive nodes (stage II, III) or metastases (stage IV)
  - Some experts advocate no pregnancy following invasive cancer
  - Others advocate waiting 5 years before subsequent pregnancies

Treatment
- Modified radical mastectomy and lymph node biopsy/dissection
  - Traditional treatment if pregnancy not interrupted
  - For stage I, stage II and some stage III
  - Obviates need for radiation (harmful to fetus)
  - Sentinel lymph node requires isotope (possibly harmful)
- Breast conservation becoming increasingly more common
  - Late 2nd or 3rd trimester can perform lumpectomy
    - Chemotherapy can be given after 1st trimester
    - Radiation therapy can be given after delivery
- Radiotherapy avoided during all trimesters
  - Due to dose absorbed by fetus
- Chemotherapy and tamoxifen avoided during first trimester
  - Due to risk of fetal damage
- Therapeutic abortion not proven to improve survival

Prognosis
- Survival equal stage by stage to non-pregnancy-related carcinoma
- Overall has worse prognosis due to more advanced presentation

Selected References
1. Woo JC et al: Breast cancer in pregnancy: A literature review. Arch Surg 138:91-8, 2003
2. Gemignani ML et al: Breast cancer during pregnancy: Diagnostic and therapeutic dilemmas. Adv Surg 34:273-86, 2000
3. Liberman L et al: Imaging of pregnancy-associated breast cancer. Radiology 191:245-8, 1994

Pregnancy

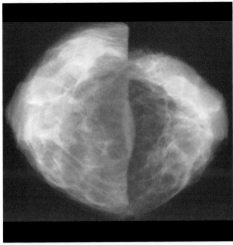

Pregnancy. 33-year-old pregnant woman with normal mammogram. Bilateral CC view.

Key Facts
- Most common benign breast lesions diagnosed during pregnancy
  - Fibroadenoma, lipoma, papilloma, fibrocystic changes, galactocele, inflammatory changes, lactating adenoma
- Pregnancy affects breast cancer risk
  - Least in women with first pregnancy before age 30
  - Intermediate with first pregnancy after age 30
  - Greatest in women who have never been pregnant
  - Miscarriage or abortion may increase risk (controversial)
- Breast cancer most frequent malignancy in pregnancy
  - Incidence: 1:3,000 - 1:10,000
  - Average age: mid-to-late thirties
- Breast biopsy in pregnancy
  - No contraindication to core needle biopsy or fine needle aspirate (FNA)
    - FNA specimens in benign pregnant breast tissue extremely cellular
    - Difficult to differentiate from malignancy
    - Core biopsy more reliable
  - Caution with surgical biopsy
    - Careful attention to hemostasis
    - Local anesthesia preferred

Imaging Findings
Mammography Findings
- Bilateral and symmetrical increase in radiographic density
  - Proliferation of confluent nodular densities
  - Loss of surrounding contrasting fatty tissue
- Mammographic changes may limit sensitivity and diagnostic value
  - Takes 3-6 months after delivery for mammographic changes to resolve
  - Mammography recommended only if clinical circumstances extremely suspicious or ultrasound findings equivocal
    - Masses may be obscured by increased radiodensity

Pregnancy

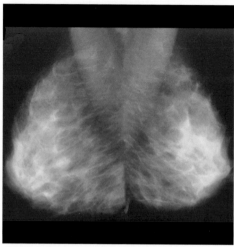

Pregnancy. 33-year-old pregnant woman with normal mammogram. Bilateral MLO view.

- ▪ Ca++ may be detected even in extremely dense tissue
  - o Abdomen should be shielded with lead apron
    - ▪ Without shield most radiation absorbed by maternal soft tissues
    - ▪ Virtually no radiation reaches fetus
- Radiation Risks
  - o Embryo death
    - ▪ Peri-implantation period (conception to 10-14 days)
  - o Congenital malformations
    - ▪ Organogenesis (days 10-14 through eighth week)
  - o Intrauterine growth retardation, low birth weight
    - ▪ Fetal period (eight weeks to term)
  - o Post-natal neoplasia
    - ▪ Theoretical risk; controversial
- Interruption of pregnancy not recommended by American College of Radiology for exposures less than 5 cGy

Ultrasound Findings
- Echogenicity usually decreased in pregnancy
- Echo pattern
  - o Homogeneous; finely granular
- Late pregnancy
  - o Lactiferous ducts distended
    - ▪ Hypoechoic to anechoic tubular structures

MR Findings
- Not indicated in pregnancy
  - o Significant generalized contrast enhancement
    - ▪ Identification of malignant processes difficult

Imaging Recommendations
- Ultrasound

Pregnancy

Differential Diagnosis: Imaging and Pathological
Hormone Replacement Therapy
Lactation
- Pregnancy-like change
- Occurs in patients who are neither pregnant nor lactating
- Affects pre- or post-menopausal women who have been pregnant in the past
- Occasionally seen in men treated with estrogen
- Breast lobules resemble those in pregnancy and lactation

Pathology
- Early pregnancy (1st trimester)
  - Rapid growth of terminal ducts and lobules = lobular enlargement
  - Depletion of fibrofatty stroma and increased stromal vascularity
  - Infiltration of mononuclear inflammatory cells
- Mid to late pregnancy
  - Progressive lobular growth
    - Cellular enlargement and proliferation
  - Vacuolated cytoplasm of lobular epithelial cells
  - Accumulation of secretions in distended lobules
  - Nuclei hyperchromatic
    - Small nucleoli
- Electron microscopy
  - Flattened, attenuated myoepithelial cells
  - Organelle-rich cytoplasm
  - Prominent endoplasmic reticulum
  - Swollen mitochondria
- Estrogen/Progesterone Receptors (ER/PR) of malignant tumors more often negative than in non-pregnant age-matched controls

Clinical Issues
Presentation
- Breast enlargement, pain
- Hyperpigmentation of areola and nipple
- Dilated cutaneous veins
- Small amount of colostrum production
Prognosis
- Worse prognosis for breast cancer diagnosed in pregnancy
  - Result of delay in diagnosis
  - Malignant lesions may be obscured by generalized lumpiness of pregnancy
  - Tumors larger, later stage
  - More frequent vascular invasion
  - Axillary node metastasis 60-70%

Selected References
1. Swinford AE et al: Mammographic appearance of the breasts during pregnancy and lactation: False assumptions. Acad Radiol 5(7): 467-72, 1998
2. Petrek AP: Breast cancer in pregnancy. Breast Diseases. 2nd edition:809-12. 1991
3. Gregl A et al: The diagnostic value of mammography during pregnancy and lactation. Rofo: Fortschritte auj dem Gebiete der Rentgenstrahlen ud der Nuklearmedizin 127(6): 535-40, 1977

PocketRadiologist®
Breast
Top 100 Diagnoses

PROCEDURES

Fine Needle Aspiration Biopsy

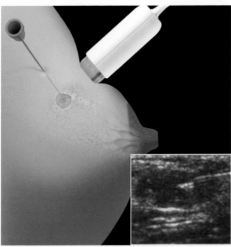

Accurate fine needle aspiration depends on optimal positioning of the transducer in relation to the target and the needle. The long axis of the transducer should be parallel to the needle shaft and focused on the area to be biopsied. The insert reflects the expected image when such positioning is achieved.

Key Facts
- Synonym: Fine needle aspiration (FNA)
- Definition: Aspiration of cells from solid masses
- Clinical setting triggering procedure
  - Palpable mass
  - Image detected mass
- Best procedure approach
  - 21-gauge or smaller needle attached to syringe
    - May use small needle without syringe ("syphon" method)
  - As samples are taken, suction is applied by way of syringe
  - Needle excursion is an advance/retract shearing motion
  - Needle tip angle should be altered to sample a broad region of mass
- Most feared complication
  - A fairly benign invasive procedure
  - Inadequate sampling results in necessity for rebiopsy
- Expected outcome
  - Obtain cellular aspirate for cytologic interpretation
  - Findings should affect clinical management recommendations
- Procedure requires facility to have excellent cytopathologists

Pre-Procedure
Indications
- Clinically worrisome mass
- Image-detected suspicious mass
Contraindications (Relative)
- Lack of adequately trained cytopathologists limits interpretation accuracy
- Not recommended for aspiration of calcifications
Getting Started
- Things to check
  - Mass must be visible on imaging modality directing procedure

Fine Needle Aspiration Biopsy

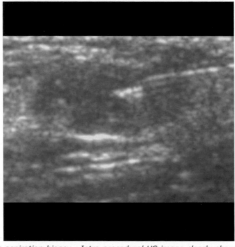

Fine needle aspiration biopsy. Intra-procedural US image clearly shows needle tip within a hypoechoic mass. Fine needle aspiration revealed cells diagnostic of fibroadenoma.

- Equipment List
  - When applicable, US is the imaging modality of choice
    - \> 7 MHz linear transducer
    - Experienced imager with interventional experience
  - Mammographic units including stereotactic prone tables may be used
  - MRI FNA is performed at some facilities
  - Needles and syringes
  - Slides

Procedure
<u>Patient Position, Location</u>
- Patient is in supine or a rolled position for US-guided FNA
<u>Equipment Preparation</u>
- Transducer may be covered with clear plastic wrap or with a sterile sleeve
- Betadine may be used as the coupling agent
  - Alternatively sterile gel is used
<u>Procedure Steps</u>
- Focused area is cleaned in a standard sterile fashion
- Local anesthesia
  - A small amount of bicarbonate added to 1% lidocaine to ↓ burning sensation
- US guidance is used throughout procedure
- Needle is introduced into mass
- A to-and-fro, or shearing motion with constant negative pressure allows cells to be collected into needle
  - 10-15 to-and-fro motions of the needle fanning out to sample different areas suggested
- Suction is released before removing needle from mass
- Needle is removed from syringe, air is sucked into syringe and needle reattached

Fine Needle Aspiration Biopsy

- Material in needle is gently pushed out onto slides
  - Slides may be air dried or fixed
  - Important to communicate method to cytologist
- Residual material may be placed into special solutions
  - These preparations are centrifuged creating a button of cells for cytologic evaluation

Alternative Procedures, Therapies
- Radiologic
  - Core biopsy with image guidance
    - Does not require additional cytopathology expertise
    - Provides histologic rather than just cellular information
    - +/- invasion
    - Tumor marker evaluation possible/more accurate

Surgical
- Lesion may be excised
  - By palpation
  - With image-guided pre-surgical needle localization

Post-Procedure
Things to Do
- Prepare slides per pathology laboratory protocol
- Tell patient possible late complications and actions to take
  - Bleeding or infection

Common Problems & Complications
Problems
- Bloody aspirates may limit sampling
- Small, blood-filled lesions may disappear
- Consider placing a clip at the site to direct surgical excision

Complications
- Vasovagal reactions
  - Very uncommon when patient is supine or prone
  - Possible when patient upright as in add-on stereotactic mammography unit
- Bleeding
  - Very uncommon with this procedure
- Infection
  - Very uncommon

Selected References
1. Daniel BL et al: Freehand iMRI-guided large-gauge core needle biopsy; a new minimally invasive technique for diagnosis of enhancing breast lesions. J Mag Reson Imaging 13:896-902, 2001
2. Cardenosa G: Breast Imaging Companion. Lippincott-Raven, Philadelphia PA, pp 384, 1997
3. Dowlatshahi K et al: Nonpalpable breast lesions: Findings of sterotaxic needle-core biopsy and fine-needle aspiration cytology. Radiology 181:745-50, 1991

Galactography

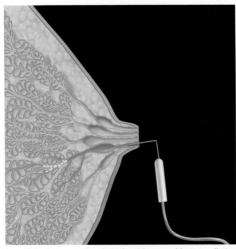

Galactography. If discharge can be elicited, a 30-gauge blunt needle is placed within the discharging duct and contrast slowly injected. Depicted here is a filling defect (oval white material) within a branch of the injected duct (blue-filled areas).

Key Facts
- Procedure synonym: Ductogram
- Procedure definition: Contrast injection of discharging duct followed by mammographic images
- Clinical setting triggering procedure – spontaneous nipple discharge
- Best procedure approach
  - Direct visualization of discharging duct orifice followed by cannulation with a small, blunt-tipped needle
- Most feared complication
  - Contrast reaction (very rare)
- Expected outcome
  - Contrast-filled ductal system may demonstrate filling defect causing nipple discharge
  - Findings direct follow-up recommendations

Pre-Procedure
Indications
- Spontaneous single duct nipple discharge

Contraindications
- Mastitis

Getting Started
- Must be able to elicit nipple discharge
  - Typically focus on only one discharging duct
  - Can do additional duct injections
    - May lead to ambiguity
    - Arborizing ductal systems may overlap and obscure filling defects
- Equipment List
  - Mammography unit
  - 30-gauge blunt-ended, sialography needle attached to flexible tubing
  - 1-3 cc Luer-Lok syringe

Galactography

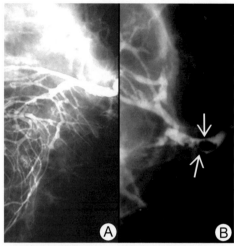

Galactography. (A) Normal galactogram (B) Patient with spontaneous bloody nipple discharge had a single discharging duct cannulated and injected with water-soluble contrast. Lateral magnification galactogram demonstrating a central ductal filling defect (arrows). Surgery found a papilloma.

- o Undiluted iodinated water-soluble contrast
- o Use care to eliminate all air bubbles

Procedure
<u>Patient Position, Location</u>
- May be supine or sitting upright
- Typically performed near mammography unit

<u>Equipment Preparation</u>
- Set up the mammography unit for magnification views

<u>Procedure Steps</u>
- Discharge must be visible at offending duct orifice
- The nipple is cleansed in a standard sterile fashion
- Xylocaine jelly may be applied to decrease nipple sensation
- A magnifying device may aide in visualization of the tiny duct orifice
- The discharging duct is cannulated with blunt needle
  - o No force should be applied
  - o Needle insertion typically painless
- 0.2-0.4 cc water soluble contrast slowly introduced
- The injection is stopped when patient perceives breast fullness
  - o Terminate injection if there is sharp pain
    - ▪ May indicate extravasation
- The needle is taped in place
  - o Allows additional injection if necessary
- Magnified full paddle CC and lateral mammogram is taken

<u>Alternative Procedures, Therapies</u>
- Ultrasound
  - o Sonography of the subareolar area
    - ▪ May demonstrate dilated duct with visible filling defect
- MRI

Galactography

- Surgical
  - Endoscopic imaging
  - Duct exploration

Post-Procedure
Things To Do
- No specific requirements
- May aspirate contrast-nipple discharge for cytology
  - Very low yield
- If intraductal lesion is diagnosed
  - May perform preoperative galactogram
  - 1:1 methylene blue and contrast
  - Orthogonal galactogram views direct needle localization

Common Problems & Complications
Problems
- Difficulties in duct cannulation
  - Hot towel over nipple
  - Manually elongate nipple to straighten duct
- Air bubbles inadvertently injected may be mistaken for lesions
- Over-injection may cause peripheral extravasation
Complications
- Severe
  - Contrast reaction
  - Very rare
- Other complications
  - Duct perforation (rare)
  - Trauma to duct from procedure
  - Injection into vein (rare)
  - Disruption of duct secondary to cancer
- May repeat procedure same day after contrast reabsorbed

Selected References
1. Orel SG et al: MI imaging in patients with nipple discharge: Initial experience. Radiology 216:248-54, 2000
2. Kopans D: Breast imaging 2nd edition. Lippincott-Raven, Philadelphia PA. Chapter 21, 703-4, 1998
3. Cardenosa G: Breast imaging companion. Lippincott-Raven, Philadelphia PA, 373-83, 1997

Pre-Surgical Lesion Localization

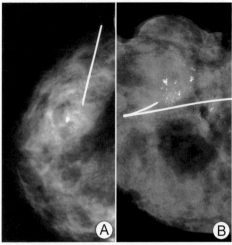

X-ray grid technique. (A) Lateral view with needle placement directed by alphanumeric grid coordinates (not shown) and a cranial caudal view with needle tip beyond the calcifications. Blue dye was injected followed by hookwire deployment. (B) Specimen x-ray with calcifications and hookwire.

Key Facts
- Procedure synonyms: Needle loc, wire placement, J-wire
- Procedure definition: Image-guided localization of non-palpable breast lesions prior to surgical excision
- Clinical setting triggering procedure: Image-detected non-palpable suspicious breast lesion recommended for surgical excision
- Best procedure approach
  o Grid localization method for mammographic guidance
  o Free-hand approach for sonographic guidance
  o Free-hand or modified grid approach for MRI guidance
- Most feared complication(s)
  o Vasovagal response
  o Inaccurate localization
  o Wire migration
- Expected outcome
  o Target accurately localized with a marking wire(s)
  o Accurate surgical removal of target and marking wire(s)
  o Verification of target and wire removal by specimen imaging

Pre-Procedure
<u>Indications</u>
- Following percutaneous core biopsy cancer diagnosis
- Some high-risk non-cancer lesions
  o Atypical hyperplasias
  o Lobular neoplasias
- Other non-cancer lesions (more controversial)
  o Papillary lesions
  o Cellular epithelial lesions
  o Radial scars

Pre-Surgical Lesion Localization

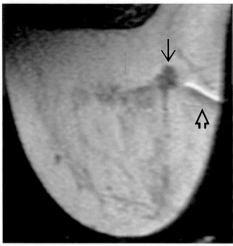

Axial T1 C- MR image during pre-operative needle localization procedure demonstrates a spiculated lesion (arrow) and the artifact from the localization needle (open arrow). Free-hand localization relies on incremental needle advancement and sequential imaging.

- Certain lesions may warrant consideration of surgical excision as initial biopsy method (practice specific)
  - Architectural distortion
  - Some broadly distributed calcifications

Contraindications
- No specific contraindications

Getting Started
- Target lesion must be clearly visible on imaging modality used to guide procedure
- Guidance choice factors
  - Equipment available
  - Lesion location
  - Ease of patient positioning
  - Experience of radiologist
- Equipment list
  - Mammographic unit
    - Alphanumeric grid-adapted compression paddle
  - Prone table stereotactic unit for stereotactic localization
  - Mammographic unit add-on stereotactic device
  - Sonographic machine
    - Requires at least a 7 MHz linear transducer
  - MRI
    - Dedicated breast coil
    - MRI-compatible needles
    - Expertise in diagnostic gadolinium-enhanced breast MRI
    - Open or closed bore magnets

Pre-Surgical Lesion Localization

Procedure

Patient Position, Location
- Mammographic localization
  - Patient sitting
  - May recline on gurney or special procedure chair
- Sonographic localization
  - Patient supine or rolled
- MRI localization
  - Patient prone on breast coil

Equipment Preparation
- Sterile localization needle
- Local anesthetic
- Betadine or other accepted sterile cleansing agent

Procedure Steps
- Image guidance provided for needle placement at or through lesion
- May inject 0.1-0.4 cc methylene blue into targeted tissue area
- More than one localization needle may be used to surround lesion
- Secure wire to patient skin with tape
  - No tension should be applied as this may dislodge hookwire
- Unilateral mammogram verifies final wire placement
  - Regardless of image guidance used, unilateral mammogram suggested
  - Helpful to surgeon to direct approach and depth
- Intraoperative specimen imaging verifies lesion and wire removal
  - X-ray, sonographic
  - Findings phoned directly to operating surgeon

Alternative Procedures, Therapies
- Radiological Procedure
  - Percutaneous image-guided core biopsy may eliminate need for surgical biopsy in many lesions
- Surgical Procedure
  - Clinically apparent lesions may not require image-guided localization

Post-Procedure

Things to Do
- Mark post-procedural mammogram films
  - Lesion and methylene blue injection sites
- Speak directly to surgeon for complicated cases

Things to Avoid
- Incomplete imaging workup prior to procedure date

Common Problems & Complications

Problems
- Lesion no longer visible on day of procedure

Complications
- Vasovagal reaction
  - Typically responds to conservative treatment
- Infection or significant bleeding very rare

Selected References
1. Daniel BL, et al: Breast lesion localization: A freehand, interactive MR imaging-guided technique. Radiology 207:455-463, 1998
2. de Paredes ES et al: Interventional breast procedures. Curr Probl Diagn Radiol 27:133-84, 1998
3. Bassett LW et al: Diagnosis of diseases of the breast. WB Saunders Co, Philadelphia PA; Chapter 16, 243-50, 1997

Sentinel Lymph Node Mapping

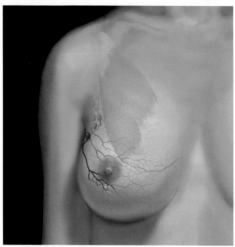

Schematic representation of intraoperatively injected isosulfan blue dye uptake by the lymphatic channels leading to the sentinel lymph node. A few minutes following peritumoral (or retroareolar) injection, an axillary incision is made and the blue channels/lymph nodes visually identified and dissected.

Key Facts
- Procedure synonyms: Sentinel lymph node biopsy (SLNB)
- Procedure definition: Identification of initial sentinel lymph node(s) (SLN) draining known breast tumor using radiocolloid, isosulfan blue dye, or both
- Clinical setting triggering procedure
  - Invasive cancers
  - Extensive ductal carcinoma in situ (DCIS)
- Best procedure approach
  - Greatest operative SLN identification success when both mapping agents are used
- Most feared complication
  - Anaphylactic reaction to isosulfan blue dye injection
- Expected outcome
  - Audible and/or direct visual identification of SLN by surgeon
  - SLN dissected out
  - Extensive histologic evaluation
  - Limits need for full axillary dissection

Pre-Procedure
Indications
- Invasive tumors
- Extensive DCIS
Contraindications (Relative)
- Recommendations are changing
- Initial concerns
  - Large tumors
  - Large post lumpectomy sites
  - Post-neoadjuvant chemotherapy

314

Sentinel Lymph Node Mapping

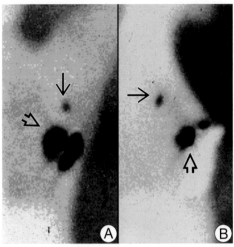

Sentinel lymph node mapping. Frontal (A) and lateral (B) lymphoscintigraphy views following peritumoral radiocolloid injection (arrowheads) show a single axillary SLN (arrows).

  o Abnormal clinical axillary examination
<u>Getting Started</u>
- Equipment List
  o Nuclear medicine gamma camera
    ▪ If performing lymphoscintigraphy
  o Hand-held gamma probe
    ▪ Used by surgeon for audible intraoperative SLN identification

Procedure
<u>Patient Position, Location</u>
- Patient supine
- Radiocolloid injection typically in nuclear medicine department hours before surgery
- Isosulfan blue dye injected intraoperatively by surgeon
<u>Procedure Steps</u>
- Radiocolloid injection
  o Many techniques
    ▪ Greatest experience = peritumoral
    ▪ Intradermal injections may not visualize internal mammary nodes
  o Varying doses
    ▪ 3.7 – 111 MBq
  o Varying volumes of saline
    ▪ 0.1 – 5 ml
  o Varying numbers of injections
    ▪ Single – 3 or more
    ▪ Spaced 1 cm apart
  o Varying time intervals between injection and surgery
    ▪ 2 hours – 24 hours (day before surgery)
    ▪ Longer wait = increased likelihood of SLN visualization on lymphoscintigraphy

- ▪ Smaller particles may progress more rapidly than larger particles
- Lymphoscintigraphy
  - o Most SLNs are imaged with this technique; few are not visualized
  - o May direct surgeon to internal mammary as well as axillary SLN
  - o May direct SLN wire localization by radiologist prior to surgical excision
  - o Not required for audible intraoperative SLN identification
- Intraoperative procedure
  - o Hand-held gamma probe identifies radioactive SLN
    - ▪ Directs surgical dissection
  - o Direct intraoperative injection of isosulfan blue dye
    - ▪ Volume based on patient size
    - ▪ 1-5 ml
    - ▪ Rapid uptake
    - ▪ Node dissection visually directed
    - ▪ Identification of blue lymphatic tracts and nodes

Alternative Procedures, Therapies
- Surgical
  - o Standard full axillary dissection

Post-Procedure
Things to Do
- Extensive histologic assessment of SLN
- Frozen section evaluation
  - o If positive, continue full axillary dissection
  - o If negative, wait for standard histology evaluation
- Standard hematoxylin & eosin histology evaluation
  - o If positive
    - ▪ Full axillary dissection (levels I and II)
  - o If negative
    - ▪ Consider immunohistochemical evaluation
- Axillary nodal histology positive
  - o Systemic treatment typically recommended

Common Problems & Complications
Problems
- Difficulty in intraoperative SLN identification
  - o Surgeon's statistics improve with experience
Complications
- Severe
  - o Anaphylactic shock following isosulfan blue injection

Selected References
1. Schwartz GF et al: Proceedings of the consensus conference on the role of sentinel lymph node biopsy in carcinoma of the breast April 19-22, 2001, Philadelphia, PA, USA. The Breast Journal 8:126-8, 2002
2. Birdwell RL et al: Breast cancer variables affecting sentinel lymph node visualization at preoperative lymphoscintigraphy. Radiology 220:47-53, 2001
3. Liberman L et al: Percutaneous biopsy and sentinel lymphadenectoomy: Minimally invasive diagnosis and treatment of nonpalpable breast cancer. AJR 177:887-91, 2001

Stereotactic Biopsy

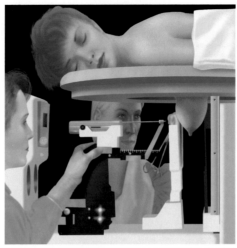

Stereotactic biopsy. The hydraulic mechanism incorporated in the dedicated prone biopsy tables allows the radiologist and technologist to work on the compressed breast sitting underneath the patient.

Key Facts
- Procedure synonyms: Stereotaxic biopsy, stereo core biopsy
- Procedure definition: X-ray image-guided percutaneous needle biopsy using stereotactic equipment
- Clinical setting triggering procedure
  - Nonpalpable mammographically-detected suspicious lesions
- Best procedure approach
  - Dedicated prone table system
  - Upright add-on to mammographic unit
  - Needle choice: Vacuum-assisted single entry or tru-cut multiple entry
  - 14-8 gauge sizes available
  - 11 gauge vacuum-assisted needle often used for sampling calcifications
- Most feared complication
  - Bleeding
- Expected outcome
  - Targeted lesion adequately sampled directing follow-up recommendations

Pre-Procedure
Indications
- Both low and highly suspicious lesions may be amenable to biopsy
  - Calcifications more common target than masses
  - Some controversy concerning highly suspicious lesions
    - Referring physician and patient concern re: tumor seeding
Contraindications
- Patient inability to lie still in prone position for 30-60 minutes
- Lesion size and location and breast size may limit procedure use
Getting Started
- Full imaging workup prior to procedure
- Lesion must be clearly visible

Stereotactic Biopsy

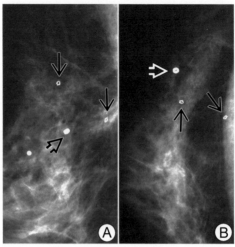

Post-stereotactic core biopsy mammogram shows 2 clips (arrows) and 1 marker (open arrows). The choice of different clip/markers benefits the patient when more than one procedure is performed by allowing more accurate identification of the areas biopsied (A = lateral and B = CC post biopsy mammogram).

- Equipment List
  - Dedicated prone stereotactic table
    - May choose add-on stereotactic equipment available with some mammographic units
  - 11-gauge vacuum-assisted biopsy needle
    - Most commonly used needle at this time for sampling calcifications

Procedure
Patient Position, Location
- Prone on specially designed table equipped with stereotactic imaging
- Upright with add-on mammographic unit stereotactic unit
Equipment Preparation
- Phantom targeting performed on daily basis
- Local anesthetic
  - With and without epinephrine
  - Epinephrine assists in hemostasis and prolongs anesthesia
- Scalpel, 11 gauge
- Skin hook may be used
Procedure Steps
- Scout imaging verifies target
- Two stereotactic images taken
  - 15° each side of perpendicular to film plane
- Needle mounted on driver
- System directs needle entry to X & Y coordinates
  - Depth, or Z axis, calculated from parallax shift on stereo images
  - Some units move needle guide automatically to position
  - Must incorporate needle length into calculations
- Anesthesia injected
- Small skin nick made at level of needle insertion

Stereotactic Biopsy

- Needle inserted and pre-fire stereotactic images obtained
- Needle fully extended into breast ("fired")
- Post-fire stereotactic images obtained
- Lesion biopsy samples taken
- X-ray core biopsy samples to verify calcification retrieval
- May place a clip/marker to indicate region sampled
- Perform post-procedural upright mammogram
  - Establish clip position

Alternative Procedures, Therapies
- Radiologic Procedures
  - Sonographically-guided biopsy if lesion visible with this modality
  - MRI-guided biopsy may be recommended
    - If lesion(s) more clearly/only visible with this modality
- Surgical Procedures
  - Surgical excision without prior percutaneous biopsy (practice specific)
    - Architectural distortion; broadly distributed calcifications
    - Surgeon or patient preference
- Other Procedures
  - Percutaneous ablation

Post-Procedure
Things to Do
- Counsel patient as to possible late complications
  - Hematoma, infection, sampling errors
  - Possible surgical biopsy recommendation for non-malignant histology
    - Atypical hyperplasias, lobular neoplasias, radial scar, papillary lesions
- Must verify imaging/pathology concordance

Things to Avoid
- Delay in post-procedural recommendations

Common Problems & Complications
Problems
- Difficulty identifying lesion on digital small field-of-view image
- Difficulty in targeting or sampling lesions
  - Very posterior or superficial
  - Retroareolar
  - Very thin breast

Complications
- Severe
  - Uncontrolled bleeding
- Other complications
  - Inaccurate lesion sampling
  - Clip/marker not in area of biopsy
  - Infection

Selected References
1. Liberman L et al: One operation after percutaneous diagnosis of non-palpable breast cancer. AJR177:887-91, 2001
2. Liberman L: Percutaneous imaging-guided core breast biopsy: State of the art at the millennium. AJR 174:1191-9, 2000
3. Kopans D: Breast imaging 2nd edition. Lippincott-Raven, Philadelphia PA; Chapter 21, 710-15, 1998

Ultrasound-Guided Needle Biopsy

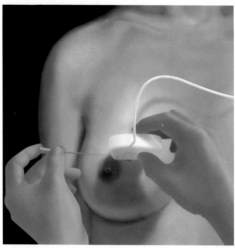

The technique for US-guided interventional procedures relies on aligning the needle parallel with the long axis of the transducer. For efficiency and expedience, the radiologist should hold the needle in his/her dominant hand and the transducer in the non-dominant hand (rather than having an assistant hold the transducer).

Key Facts
- Procedure synonyms: US fine needle aspiration (FNA), US core biopsy
- Procedure definition: Ultrasound guidance for interventional procedures
- Clinical setting triggering procedure
  - Suspicious lesions visible with ultrasound
- Best procedure approach
  - Breast imaged with hand-held ultrasound transducer
  - Lesion and needle simultaneously imaged in real time
- Most feared complications
  - Violation of the chest wall with core biopsy needle
  - Uncontrolled bleeding
- Expected outcome
  - Adequate sampling allowing cytologic or histologic lesion diagnosis

Pre-Procedure
Indications
- Suspicious lesions visible by ultrasound recommended for biopsy
  - Nonpalpable
  - Palpable
- Guidance can be provided for abscess drainage
  - Complete evacuation
  - Place indwelling catheter
Contraindications
- No specific contraindications
Getting Started
- Things to check
  - Lesion must be clearly visible by ultrasound
- Equipment list
  - Ultrasound machine
    - Linear 7.5 MHz transducer

Ultrasound-Guided Needle Biopsy

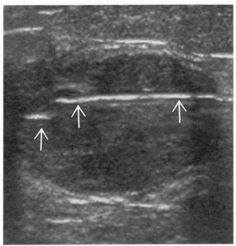

Ultrasound-guided needle biopsy. Needle (arrows) is shown within an oval well-circumscribed mass. The entire needle is clearly visible because it is parallel to the long axis of the transducer.

- Higher frequency transducer improves lesion identification
  - Biopsy needles
  - Pre-loaded clip/marker device

Procedure
Patient Position, Location
- Patient supine or obliquely placed on table next to ultrasound unit
Equipment Preparation
- Transducer must be covered
  - Non-sterile clear plastic wrap
  - Sterile sleeve
- Coupling agent
  - Betadine on skin
  - Sterile gel
- Local anesthetic
- 11 gauge scalpel
Procedure Steps
- Patient placed in a position allowing optimal lesion access
- Breast cleansed in a standard sterile fashion
- Lesion located with hand-held transducer
- Using direct real-time visualization
  - Local anesthetic injected
  - Small skin nick created
  - Biopsy needle tip moved toward lesion
    - Large lesions allow needle tip to be just inside lesion margin
    - Small lesions require needle tip just proximal to lesion
    - FNA performed with needle tip within lesion
  - Lesion sample taken
- May confirm presence of calcifications with specimen x-ray
- If entire lesion removed may choose to

Ultrasound-Guided Needle Biopsy

- o Place a clip, marker
  - Devices available for clip/marker placement through an introducer
  - Other products allow direct percutaneous marker placement

Alternative Procedures, Therapies
- Radiologic
  - o X-ray-guided biopsy if lesion visible with this modality
  - o MRI-guided biopsy may be recommended
    - If lesion(s) more clearly/only visible with this modality
- Surgical
  - o Needle-localization procedure prior to surgical excision
    - Some small lesions
    - Difficult lesion location
    - Architectural distortion
  - o Surgeon or patient preference
- Other
  - o Percutaneous ablation

Post-Procedure

Things to Do
- Counsel patient as to possible late complications
  - o Hematoma
  - o Infection
  - o Sampling errors
  - o Possible surgical biopsy recommendation for non-malignant histology
    - Atypical hyperplasias
    - Lobular neoplasias
    - Radial scar
    - Papillary lesions
- Must verify imaging/pathology concordance

Things to Avoid
- Delay in post-procedural recommendations

Common Problems & Complications

Problems
- Lesion identification
- Lesion location
  - o Deep lesions may limit biopsy needle choice
  - o Lesions adjacent to implants may limit biopsy needle choice

Complications
- Severe
  - o Penetration of chest wall with biopsy needle
  - o Uncontrolled bleeding
- Other complications
  - o Infection

Selected References
1. Fornage BD et al: Interventional breast sonography. Eur J Radiol 42:17-31, 2002
2. Liberman L: Percutaneous image-guided core breast biopsy. Radiol Clin North Am 40:483-500, 2002
3. Cardenosa G: Breast imaging companion. 391-4, 1997

Index of Diagnoses

NOTES

NOTES

NOTES

NOTES

NOTES

NOTES

NOTES

NOTES

NOTES

NOTES

NOTES

NOTES